CALM THE F*CK DOWN

A GUIDED WORKBOOK FOR ANXIETY, OVERTHINKING, AND EVERYDAY FREAK-OUTS

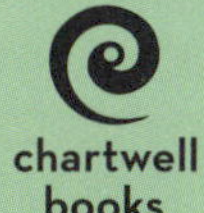

chartwell books

Contents

INTRODUCTION

Having anxiety is a completely normal experience, especially in our modern world. We have deadlines to meet, work schedules to keep up with, and dealing with the trauma of these uncertain times. All of these factors and more can contribute to the overwhelming stress that goes beyond the day-to-day. Anxiety stems from fear and feeling powerless. It's important to recognize that there's very little we have control over, but we do have control over ourselves and how we deal with what makes us anxious. You're much more powerful than you think, and you can successfully manage the stress you deal with. By becoming aware of what your triggers are, celebrating your wins, and brainstorming solutions, you can achieve inner peace and live a life unbeholden to fear.

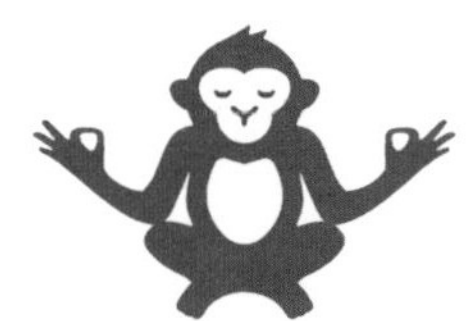

How to Use This Journal

Within these pages, you'll find mood and wellness trackers to show how your feelings change over time. They'll track your physical activity, your water intake, your overall sleep quality, and anxiety levels. These tools are here to illuminate how all these factors affect your overall mental wellbeing. You'll also find plenty of exercises to teach you how to identify your triggers, discover coping mechanisms that can prevent you from feeling overwhelmed, and a space to reflect on what you're thankful for.

For each section there will be fill in the blank portions for you to self-reflect. It's important to be honest about what you're feeling. Addressing triggers can be, in and of itself, triggering, but if you can't look at your problems, there's little hope of addressing them. Be patient with yourself as you work through your emotions, and remember, you're already taking the right steps to a more peaceful state of mind. The prompts are there to guide you. You can do this.

PRE-JOURNAL CHECK-IN

Before we jump into the hard work, let's figure out where you are today. This section is all about tracking the now. This is the beginning of your journey and will be the marker where you can see how much you've grown.

WHAT'S ON YOUR MIND? THIS CAN MEAN WHAT YOU'RE THINKING OF RIGHT THIS SECOND OR ANY RECURRING THOUGHTS THAT HAVE PLAGUED YOU TODAY.

WHAT DO YOU HOPE FOR WITH THIS JOURNAL?

ARE THERE ANY TRANSFORMATIONS YOU WANT TO SEE?

ANY SPECIFIC GOALS YOU'D LIKE TO REACH?

HOW ARE YOU FEELING? CIRCLE OR FILL IN ONE.

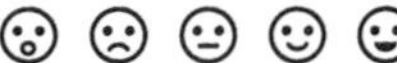

Date: ....

WELLNESS TRACKER

Here's where you'll document the physical aspects of your life that might influence your mental health.

IRRITABILITY

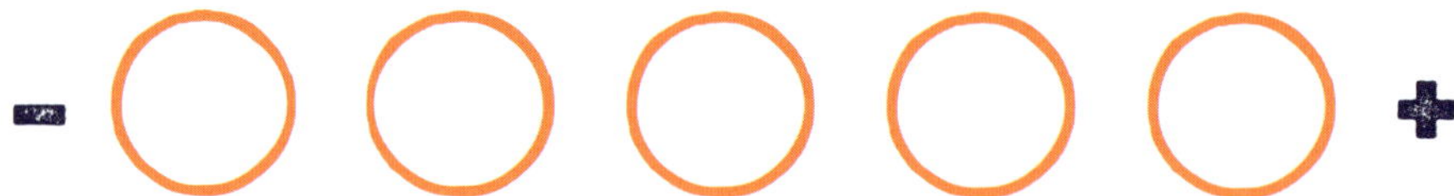

QUALITY OF SLEEP

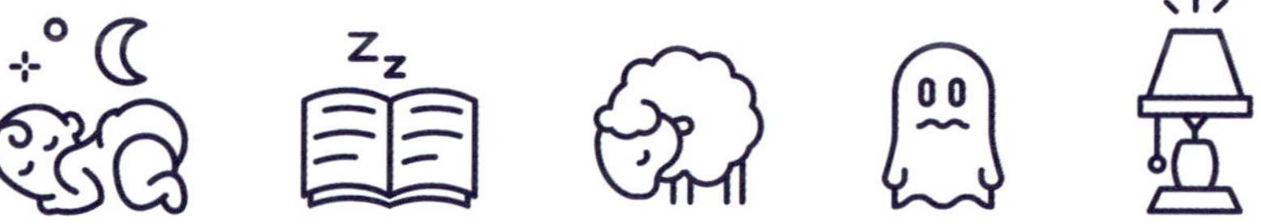

WATER INTAKE

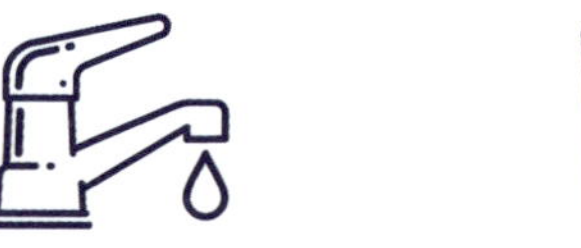

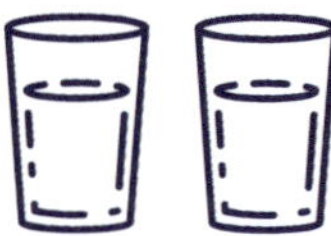

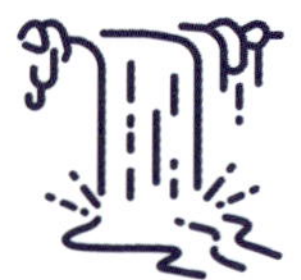

ANXIETY

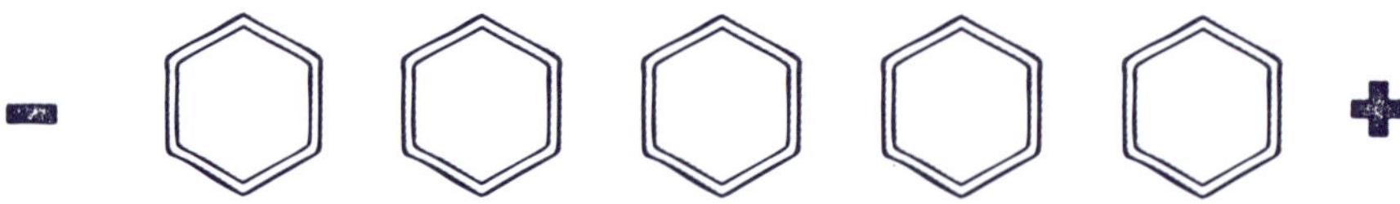

HOURS SLEPT											
-	1	2	3	4	5	6	7	8	9	10	+

HAPPY HABIT TRACKER							
HABIT TO TRACK:	S	M	T	W	TH	F	S

MEDICATION	HOW MUCH	DAY/TIME

HOW ARE YOU FEELING? CIRCLE OR FILL IN ONE.

Date: ....

WELLNESS TRACKER

Here's where you'll document the physical aspects of your life that might influence your mental health.

IRRITABILITY

- 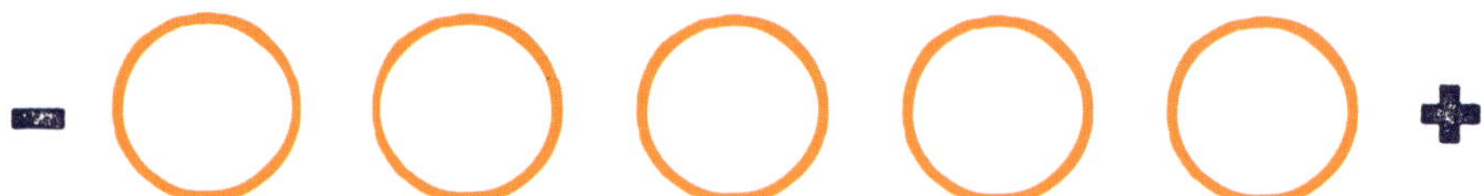 +

QUALITY OF SLEEP

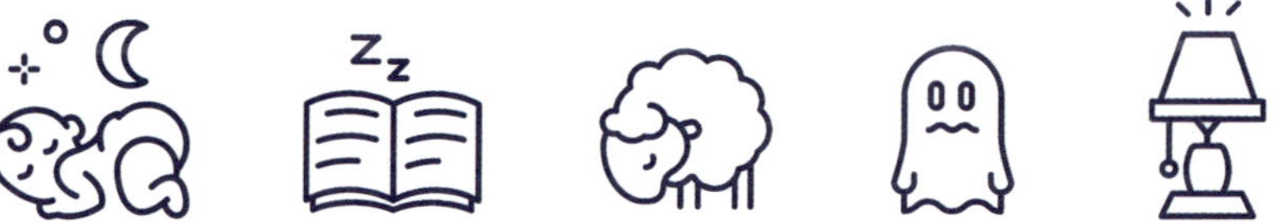

WATER INTAKE

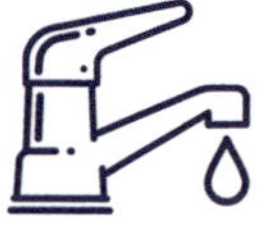

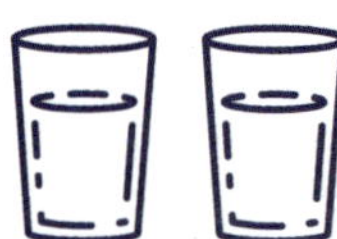

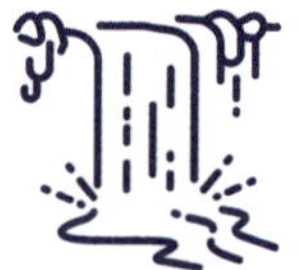

ANXIETY

- 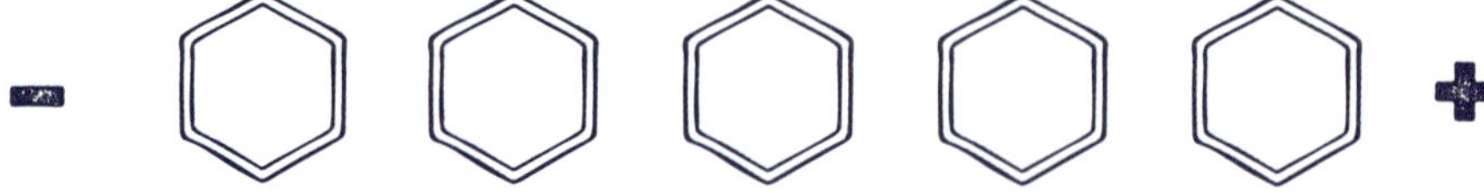 +

HOURS SLEPT											
-	1	2	3	4	5	6	7	8	9	10	+

HAPPY HABIT TRACKER

HABIT TO TRACK:	S	M	T	W	TH	F	S

MEDICATION	HOW MUCH	DAY/TIME

HOW ARE YOU FEELING? CIRCLE OR FILL IN ONE.

Date: ....

WELLNESS TRACKER

Here's where you'll document the physical aspects of your life that might influence your mental health.

IRRITABILITY

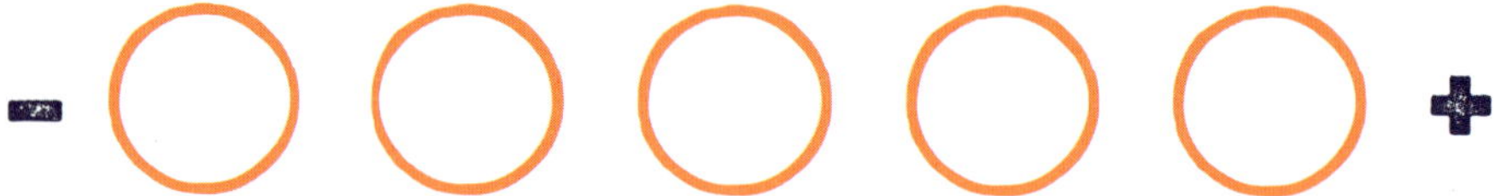

QUALITY OF SLEEP

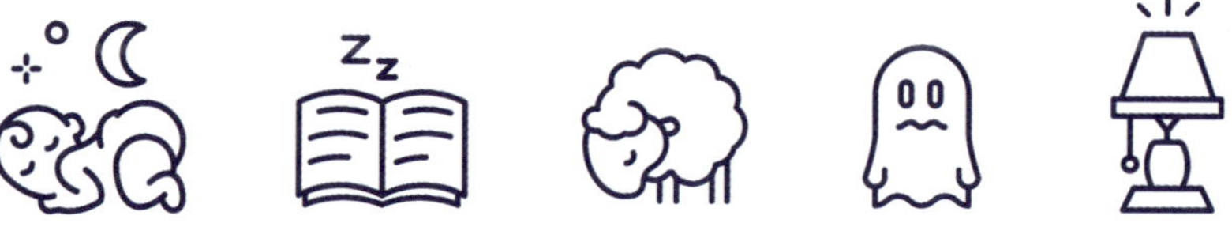

WATER INTAKE

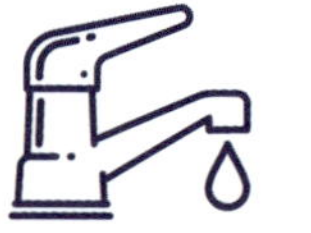

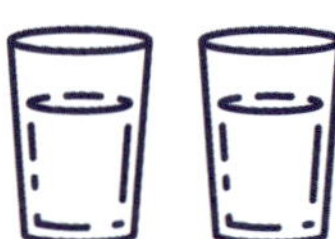

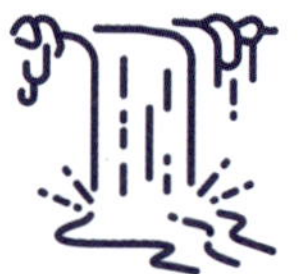

ANXIETY

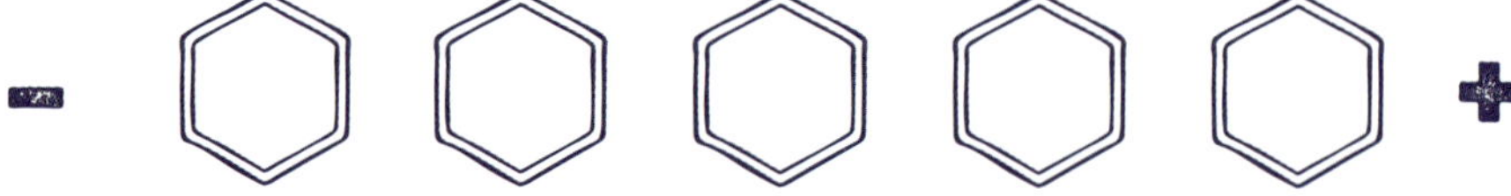

HOURS SLEPT											
-	1	2	3	4	5	6	7	8	9	10	+

HAPPY HABIT TRACKER							
HABIT TO TRACK:	S	M	T	W	TH	F	S

MEDICATION	HOW MUCH	DAY/TIME

HOW ARE YOU FEELING? CIRCLE OR FILL IN ONE.

Date: ....

WELLNESS TRACKER

Here's where you'll document the physical aspects of your life that might influence your mental health.

IRRITABILITY

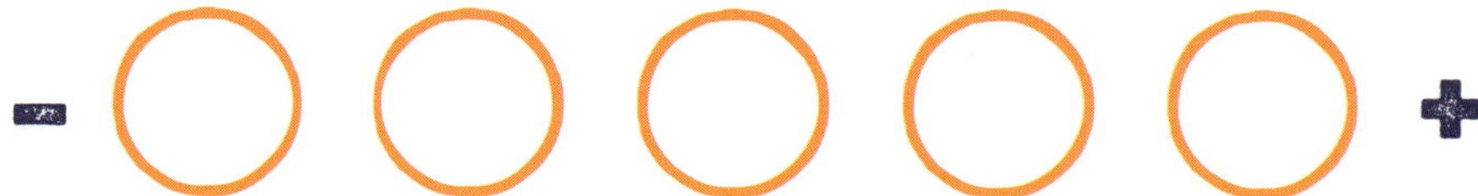

QUALITY OF SLEEP

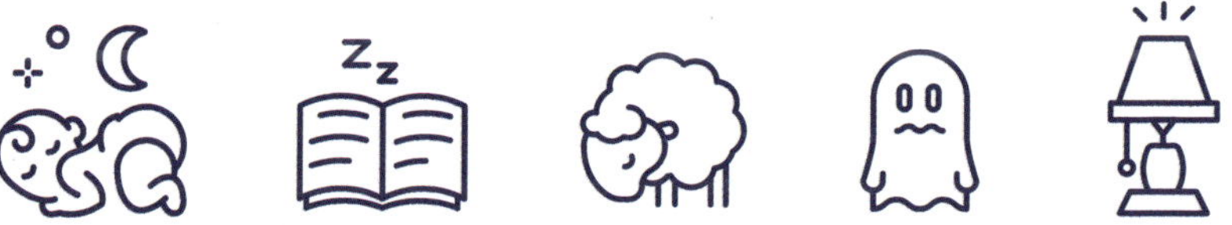

WATER INTAKE

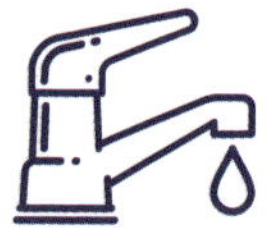

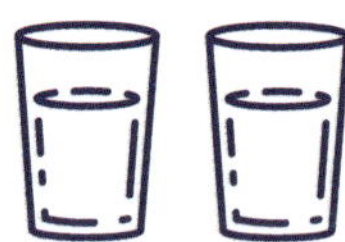

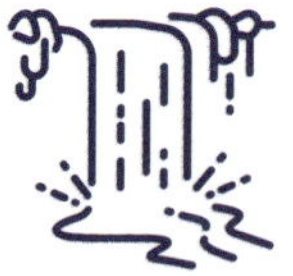

ANXIETY

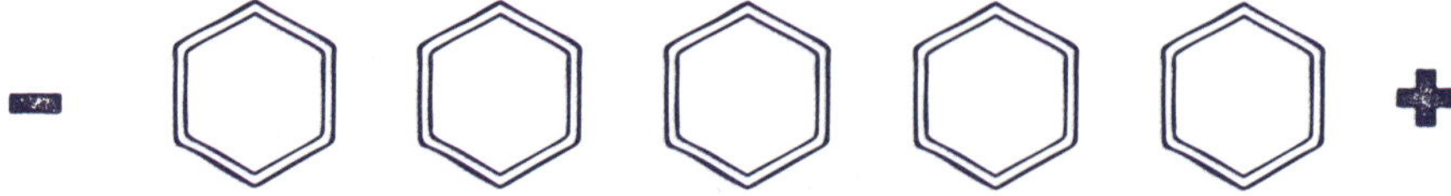

HOURS SLEPT											
-	1	2	3	4	5	6	7	8	9	10	+

HAPPY HABIT TRACKER							
HABIT TO TRACK:	**S**	**M**	**T**	**W**	**TH**	**F**	**S**

MEDICATION	HOW MUCH	DAY/TIME

HOW ARE YOU FEELING? CIRCLE OR FILL IN ONE.

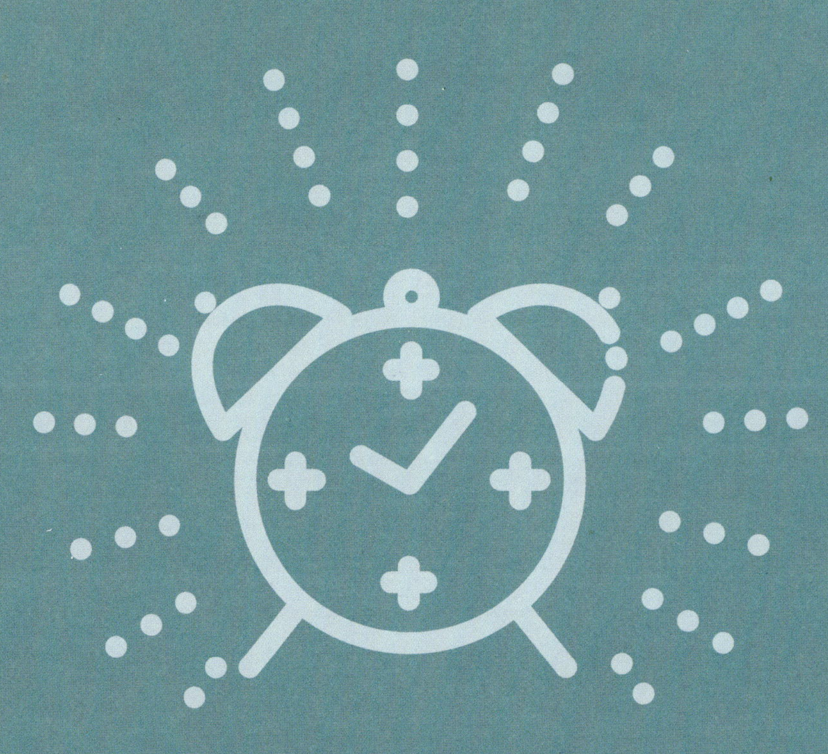

TRACKERS & TRIGGERS

When it comes to mental health, a trigger is defined as something that affects your emotional state, often in a negative way. It can take the form of pretty much anything: colors, sounds, songs, textures, words, or situations. Anxiety triggers can make a person spiral as one thought leads to another and then fear and hopelessness take over. Suddenly you have no control over yourself or anything around you. But though your thoughts and feelings may seem true, they aren't always based in reality. It's important to understand what's triggering you so you can pull back and catch yourself before you spin out.

In this section, you'll work on what makes you stressed or worried, which thought patterns take you there, what your worst fears are, and how to look at them from an objective standpoint. Once you've identified them, you'll be able to see what makes you panic and take back control. You can face them because you are stronger than your worst fears.

THOUGHT LOG

The mind is truly a powerful muscle. Left to run wild, it can conjure up all kinds of scenarios that likely won't happen. But what they will do is contribute to stress. Logging what kinds of thoughts, you're having and where they might get out of hand will provide some clarity on what causes the spiral. Once you can identify that, you can alter your thought patterns for the better.

WHEN YOU'RE STRESSED, WHAT'S THE FIRST THING THAT COMES TO MIND?

WHAT'S THE SECOND THOUGHT?

WHAT'S THE THIRD?

DO YOU FEEL OUT OF CONTROL? WHY OR WHY NOT?

JUST AS YOUR THOUGHTS CAN GET CARRIED AWAY, YOU CAN BRING THEM BACK TO YOU. HOW WILL YOU DO THIS?

HOW ARE YOU FEELING? CIRCLE ONE.

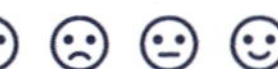

ARE YOU STRESSED? WHAT'S THE CAUSE?

WHAT WAS THE FIRST THOUGHT THAT CAME TO MIND?

WHERE DID THAT THOUGHT TAKE YOU?

AND WHERE HAVE YOU ENDED UP?

DO YOU FEEL HELPLESS? IF SO, WHERE DID THINGS GO WRONG?

HOW CAN YOU REWRITE YOUR INNER NARRATIVE TO EMPOWER YOURSELF?

WHAT'S YOUR ANXIETY LEVEL RIGHT NOW? CIRCLE ONE.

ARE YOU STRESSED? WHAT'S THE CAUSE?

WHAT WAS THE FIRST THOUGHT THAT CAME TO MIND?

WHERE DID THAT THOUGHT TAKE YOU?

AND WHERE HAVE YOU ENDED UP?

DO YOU FEEL HELPLESS? IF SO, WHERE DID THINGS GO WRONG?

HOW CAN YOU REWRITE YOUR INNER NARRATIVE TO EMPOWER YOURSELF?

WHAT'S YOUR ANXIETY LEVEL RIGHT NOW? CIRCLE ONE.

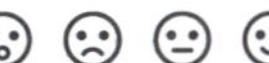

ARE YOU STRESSED? WHAT'S THE CAUSE?

WHAT WAS THE FIRST THOUGHT THAT CAME TO MIND?

WHERE DID THAT THOUGHT TAKE YOU?

AND WHERE HAVE YOU ENDED UP?

DO YOU FEEL HELPLESS? IF SO, WHERE DID THINGS GO WRONG?

HOW CAN YOU REWRITE YOUR INNER NARRATIVE TO EMPOWER YOURSELF?

WHAT'S YOUR ANXIETY LEVEL RIGHT NOW? CIRCLE ONE.

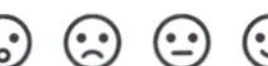

ARE YOU STRESSED? WHAT'S THE CAUSE?

WHAT WAS THE FIRST THOUGHT THAT CAME TO MIND?

WHERE DID THAT THOUGHT TAKE YOU?

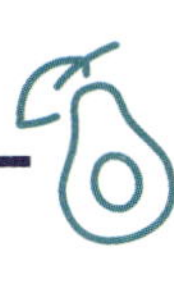

AND WHERE HAVE YOU ENDED UP?

DO YOU FEEL HELPLESS? IF SO, WHERE DID THINGS GO WRONG?

HOW CAN YOU REWRITE YOUR INNER NARRATIVE TO EMPOWER YOURSELF?

WHAT'S YOUR ANXIETY LEVEL RIGHT NOW? CIRCLE ONE.

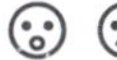   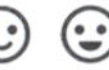

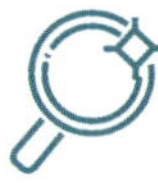

TRACKING YOUR TRIGGERS

Now that you've taken a look at your thought patterns, you can examine your triggers. What made you stressed and why? Maybe you don't know what they are yet, and that's okay. In this section you'll tackle what exactly makes you anxious, your reactions to it, and some of the thoughts that go through your mind. Whatever the trigger, it's important to identify them so you can better prepare yourself for when they appear.

DATE	TRIGGER	MOOD

DATE	TRIGGER	MOOD

WHAT'S YOUR ANXIETY LEVEL RIGHT NOW? CIRCLE ONE.

😮 ☹ 😐 🙂 😀

WHAT MAKES YOU SUPER ANXIOUS TO THE POINT THAT YOU ACTIVELY AVOID IT?

WHAT HAPPENS WHEN YOU ENCOUNTER THAT TRIGGER?

WHAT ARE SOME OF THE THOUGHTS THAT GO THROUGH YOUR MIND?

DO YOUR FEARS COMPOUND? HOW DO YOU FEEL THEN?

NAME ONE TERRIBLE THING THAT COULD HAPPEN TO YOU.

HAS IT EVER COME TRUE?

IF SO, HOW DID YOU HANDLE IT?

IF NOT, HOW LIKELY DO YOU THINK IT WILL HAPPEN? TRY TO THINK IN TERMS OF PROBABILITY AND NOT POSSIBILITY.

WHAT'S YOUR ANXIETY LEVEL RIGHT NOW? CIRCLE ONE.

IF IT'S UNLIKELY TO HAPPEN, WHAT CAN YOU THINK ABOUT INSTEAD?

IS THE TRIGGER SO SCARY NOW?

WITH SOME OF THE STING TAKEN OUT OF YOUR TRIGGER, HOW STRONG IS IT NOW?

IS YOUR ANXIETY RISING OR FALLING?

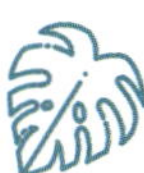

WHEN DID YOU FIRST ENCOUNTER THIS TRIGGER? WHAT HAPPENED?

WHAT ABOUT IT MAKES YOU SO ANXIOUS?

CAN YOU FORESEE YOURSELF GETTING PAST THIS?

ENVISION YOURSELF NO LONGER AFFECTED BY THIS TRIGGER. WHAT WOULD YOU DO THEN?

WHAT'S YOUR ANXIETY LEVEL RIGHT NOW? CIRCLE ONE.

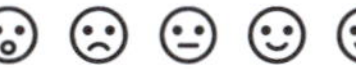

WHAT MAKES YOU SUPER ANXIOUS TO THE POINT THAT YOU ACTIVELY AVOID IT?

WHAT HAPPENS WHEN YOU ENCOUNTER THAT TRIGGER?

WHAT ARE SOME OF THE THOUGHTS THAT GO THROUGH YOUR MIND?

DO YOUR FEARS COMPOUND? HOW DO YOU FEEL THEN?

NAME ONE TERRIBLE THING THAT COULD HAPPEN TO YOU.

HAS IT EVER COME TRUE?

IF SO, HOW DID YOU HANDLE IT?

IF NOT, HOW LIKELY DO YOU THINK IT WILL HAPPEN? TRY TO THINK IN TERMS OF PROBABILITY AND NOT POSSIBILITY.

WHAT'S YOUR ANXIETY LEVEL RIGHT NOW? CIRCLE ONE.

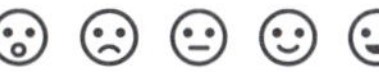

IF IT'S UNLIKELY TO HAPPEN, WHAT CAN YOU THINK ABOUT INSTEAD?

IS THE TRIGGER SO SCARY NOW?

WITH SOME OF THE STING TAKEN OUT OF YOUR TRIGGER, HOW STRONG IS IT NOW?

IS YOUR ANXIETY RISING OR FALLING?

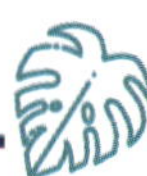

WHEN DID YOU FIRST ENCOUNTER THIS TRIGGER? WHAT HAPPENED?

WHAT ABOUT IT MAKES YOU SO ANXIOUS?

CAN YOU FORESEE YOURSELF GETTING PAST THIS?

ENVISION YOURSELF NO LONGER AFFECTED BY THIS TRIGGER. WHAT WOULD YOU DO THEN?

WHAT'S YOUR ANXIETY LEVEL RIGHT NOW? CIRCLE ONE.

WHAT MAKES YOU SUPER ANXIOUS TO THE POINT THAT YOU ACTIVELY AVOID IT?

WHAT HAPPENS WHEN YOU ENCOUNTER THAT TRIGGER?

WHAT ARE SOME OF THE THOUGHTS THAT GO THROUGH YOUR MIND?

DO YOUR FEARS COMPOUND? HOW DO YOU FEEL THEN?

NAME ONE TERRIBLE THING THAT COULD HAPPEN TO YOU.

HAS IT EVER COME TRUE?

IF SO, HOW DID YOU HANDLE IT?

IF NOT, HOW LIKELY DO YOU THINK IT WILL HAPPEN? TRY TO THINK IN TERMS OF PROBABILITY AND NOT POSSIBILITY.

WHAT'S YOUR ANXIETY LEVEL RIGHT NOW? CIRCLE ONE.

IF IT'S UNLIKELY TO HAPPEN, WHAT CAN YOU THINK ABOUT INSTEAD?

IS THE TRIGGER SO SCARY NOW?

WITH SOME OF THE STING TAKEN OUT OF YOUR TRIGGER, HOW STRONG IS IT NOW?

IS YOUR ANXIETY RISING OR FALLING?

WHEN DID YOU FIRST ENCOUNTER THIS TRIGGER? WHAT HAPPENED?

WHAT ABOUT IT MAKES YOU SO ANXIOUS?

CAN YOU FORESEE YOURSELF GETTING PAST THIS?

ENVISION YOURSELF NO LONGER AFFECTED BY THIS TRIGGER. WHAT WOULD YOU DO THEN?

WHAT'S YOUR ANXIETY LEVEL RIGHT NOW? CIRCLE ONE.

WHAT MAKES YOU SUPER ANXIOUS TO THE POINT THAT YOU ACTIVELY AVOID IT?

WHAT HAPPENS WHEN YOU ENCOUNTER THAT TRIGGER?

WHAT ARE SOME OF THE THOUGHTS THAT GO THROUGH YOUR MIND?

DO YOUR FEARS COMPOUND? HOW DO YOU FEEL THEN?

NAME ONE TERRIBLE THING THAT COULD HAPPEN TO YOU.

HAS IT EVER COME TRUE?

IF SO, HOW DID YOU HANDLE IT?

IF NOT, HOW LIKELY DO YOU THINK IT WILL HAPPEN? TRY TO THINK IN TERMS OF PROBABILITY AND NOT POSSIBILITY.

WHAT'S YOUR ANXIETY LEVEL RIGHT NOW? CIRCLE ONE.

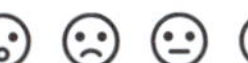

IF IT'S UNLIKELY TO HAPPEN, WHAT CAN YOU THINK ABOUT INSTEAD?

IS THE TRIGGER SO SCARY NOW?

WITH SOME OF THE STING TAKEN OUT OF YOUR TRIGGER, HOW STRONG IS IT NOW?

IS YOUR ANXIETY RISING OR FALLING?

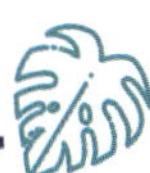

WHEN DID YOU FIRST ENCOUNTER THIS TRIGGER? WHAT HAPPENED?

WHAT ABOUT IT MAKES YOU SO ANXIOUS?

CAN YOU FORESEE YOURSELF GETTING PAST THIS?

ENVISION YOURSELF NO LONGER AFFECTED BY THIS TRIGGER. WHAT WOULD YOU DO THEN?

WHAT'S YOUR ANXIETY LEVEL RIGHT NOW? CIRCLE ONE.

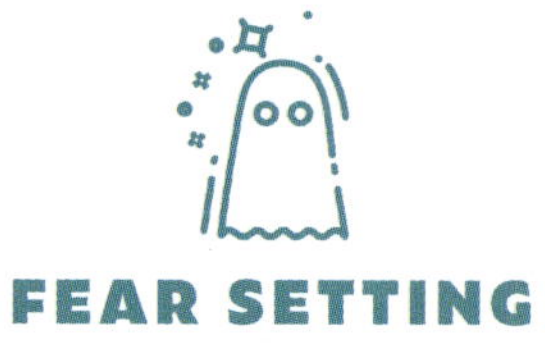

FEAR SETTING

Fear and anxiety go hand in hand. And when you're afraid, you can't see things as they really are. Instead, it's like wearing distorted goggles. But there's a way to take them off. Fear setting is an exercise where you list your fears, taking them as far as they can go, and see what can be done about them. It's about working through your fear. Are your fears likely to happen or are they just in your head? Taking an honest look into what makes your mind race will help you see if you really have anything to worry about in the first place.

In this section, you'll explore your fears, see them for what they are, and be given the tools to work through them—one page for the beginning of the week and one for the end. You'll also take a look at the warning signs for your anxiety. How do you and your body react to it? Don't forget, there's always another side to fear and you will see it. Your fears don't own you.

RIGHT OFF THE BAT, WHAT MAKES YOU NERVOUS ABOUT THIS EXERCISE, IF ANYTHING?

WHAT ARE YOU MOST EXCITED ABOUT FOR THIS EXERCISE? FINALLY CONFRONTING YOUR FEARS?

WHAT'S YOUR ANXIETY LEVEL RIGHT NOW? CIRCLE ONE.

Week of: ....

WEEKLY FEAR SETTING

WHAT ARE SOME THINGS YOU'RE NERVOUS ABOUT THIS WEEK?

HOW LIKELY WILL THESE FEARS COME TO FRUITION?

WHAT ARE SOME THINGS YOU CAN DO TO MITIGATE THE WORST POSSIBLE OUTCOME?

HOW DID THIS WEEK GO?

DID YOUR WORST FEARS COME TRUE? IF SO, HOW DID YOU HANDLE IT? IF NOT, WHAT DID YOU LEARN?

WITH THIS NEW INFORMATION, HOW WILL YOU MOVE FORWARD?

WHAT'S YOUR ANXIETY LEVEL RIGHT NOW? CIRCLE ONE.

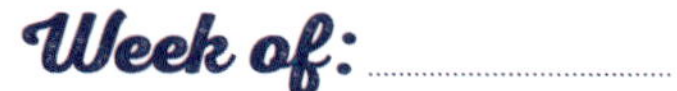

WEEKLY FEAR SETTING

WHAT ARE SOME THINGS YOU'RE NERVOUS ABOUT THIS WEEK?

HOW LIKELY WILL THESE FEARS COME TO FRUITION?

WHAT ARE SOME THINGS YOU CAN DO TO MITIGATE THE WORST POSSIBLE OUTCOME?

HOW DID THIS WEEK GO?

DID YOUR WORST FEARS COME TRUE? IF SO, HOW DID YOU HANDLE IT? IF NOT, WHAT DID YOU LEARN?

WITH THIS NEW INFORMATION, HOW WILL YOU MOVE FORWARD?

WHAT'S YOUR ANXIETY LEVEL RIGHT NOW? CIRCLE ONE.

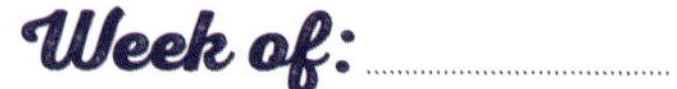

WEEKLY FEAR SETTING

WHAT ARE SOME THINGS YOU'RE NERVOUS ABOUT THIS WEEK?

HOW LIKELY WILL THESE FEARS COME TO FRUITION?

WHAT ARE SOME THINGS YOU CAN DO TO MITIGATE THE WORST POSSIBLE OUTCOME?

HOW DID THIS WEEK GO?

DID YOUR WORST FEARS COME TRUE? IF SO, HOW DID YOU HANDLE IT? IF NOT, WHAT DID YOU LEARN?

WITH THIS NEW INFORMATION, HOW WILL YOU MOVE FORWARD?

WHAT'S YOUR ANXIETY LEVEL RIGHT NOW? CIRCLE ONE.

Week of: ....

WEEKLY FEAR SETTING

WHAT ARE SOME THINGS YOU'RE NERVOUS ABOUT THIS WEEK?

HOW LIKELY WILL THESE FEARS COME TO FRUITION?

WHAT ARE SOME THINGS YOU CAN DO TO MITIGATE THE WORST POSSIBLE OUTCOME?

HOW DID THIS WEEK GO?

DID YOUR WORST FEARS COME TRUE? IF SO, HOW DID YOU HANDLE IT? IF NOT, WHAT DID YOU LEARN?

WITH THIS NEW INFORMATION, HOW WILL YOU MOVE FORWARD?

WHAT'S YOUR ANXIETY LEVEL RIGHT NOW? CIRCLE ONE.

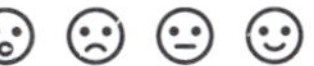

RECOGNIZING YOUR ANXIETY

Anxiety looks different for everyone. Some of the telltale signs are muscle aches, fatigue, or trembling. Documenting your body's reactions will help you become more aware of when you're feeling anxious. Then you can implement your fear setting techniques to get yourself through it.

HOW DOES YOUR BODY EXPRESS ANXIETY?

WHAT GOES THROUGH YOUR MIND? DO YOU SHUT DOWN?

WHICH SITUATIONS MAKE YOU ANXIOUS AND WHY?

WHO MAKES YOU ANXIOUS AND WHY?

WHAT MAKES YOUR ANXIETY WORSE?

WHAT'S YOUR ANXIETY LEVEL RIGHT NOW? CIRCLE ONE.

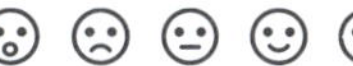

WHAT'S THE WORST THING SOMEONE CAN SAY TO YOU WHEN YOU'RE ANXIOUS AND WHY?

ARE THERE ANY NOISES THAT TRIGGER YOUR ANXIETY?

DO YOU STARTLE EASILY? IF SO, WHY? WHAT GOES THROUGH YOUR MIND?

DO YOU CONSIDER YOURSELF A PERFECTIONIST? IF SO, WHAT DRIVES YOU TO BE PERFECT?

ARE YOU ABLE TO RELAX OR DO YOU FEEL ON EDGE ALL THE TIME?

DO YOU HAVE TROUBLE SLEEPING? IF SO, HOW IS YOUR ANXIETY KEEPING YOU UP?

WHAT'S YOUR ANXIETY LEVEL RIGHT NOW? CIRCLE ONE.

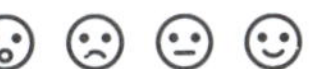

DO YOU HATE SURPRISES? IF SO, WHY?

DOES YOUR ANXIETY PREVENT YOU FROM MAKING DECISIONS?

DO YOU OVERTHINK? IN WHAT WAYS? ENVISIONING TOO MANY SCENARIOS?

DO YOU WORRY ABOUT OTHERS' OPINIONS OF YOU?

DO YOU NEED TO BE PUNCTUAL BECAUSE OF YOUR ANXIETY?

DO YOU EXPERIENCE ANXIETY ATTACKS (BOUTS OF EXTREME ANXIETY THAT ARE TYPICALLY DEBILITATING)? WHAT ARE THEY LIKE FOR YOU?

WHAT'S YOUR ANXIETY LEVEL RIGHT NOW? CIRCLE ONE.

Now that you've taken a look at how your anxieties play out, let's differentiate between your anxious self and your normal self.

DESCRIBE YOUR ANXIOUS SELF. ARE YOU ON HIGH ALERT? DOES YOUR STOMACH HURT? HOW DO YOU SEE YOURSELF?

WHAT ARE YOU LIKE WHEN YOU'RE NOT ANXIOUS? BE AS DETAILED AS POSSIBLE.

WHAT'S YOUR ANXIETY LEVEL RIGHT NOW? CIRCLE ONE.

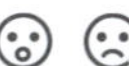   

GOODNESS & GRATITUDE

You've taken a long, hard look at your triggers and fears, you've put in the work, and now it's time to focus on the good. Anxiety can feel all-consuming, but in reality, there's so much good in the world to acknowledge. Whether it be your accomplishments, your support system, or anything else that makes you happy.

In this chapter, you'll focus on all things good to and about you. Then you'll take a look at what you're grateful for. Gratitude improves mental and physical health, cultivates empathy, and decreases resentment and frustration. With these two aspects, you're one step closer to tackling your anxiety and finding relief.

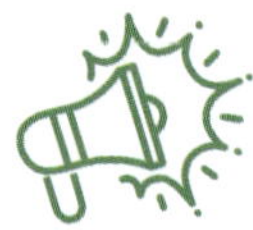

ACKNOWLEDGING YOUR ACCOMPLISHMENTS AND WINS

Sometimes the word "accomplishment" can feel like such a high standard and you might associate it with things like running a 10K or becoming valedictorian. But an accomplishment is subjective and can come in any size. As long as you overcame a challenge, it's an accomplishment.

WHAT'S AN ACHIEVEMENT YOU'RE VERY PROUD OF? WHAT MAKES THIS ONE SPECIAL?

NAME ONE OF YOUR ACHIEVEMENTS THAT YOUR LOVED ONES ARE PROUD OF AND WHY THEY'RE PROUD OF IT.

NAME ANY AWARDS YOU'VE GOTTEN OR PRIZES YOU'VE WON.

Date: ....

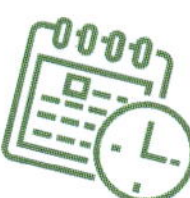

NAME THREE THINGS YOU ACCOMPLISHED TODAY, NO MATTER HOW BIG OR SMALL.

HOW DID YOU ACCOMPLISH THEM?

HOW DID YOU FEEL AFTERWARD?

LIST THE SKILLS YOU USED.

HOW ARE YOU FEELING? CIRCLE ONE.

Date: ....

NAME THREE THINGS YOU ACCOMPLISHED TODAY, NO MATTER HOW BIG OR SMALL.

HOW DID YOU ACCOMPLISH THEM?

HOW DID YOU FEEL AFTERWARD?

LIST THE SKILLS YOU USED.

Date: ....

NAME THREE THINGS YOU ACCOMPLISHED TODAY, NO MATTER HOW BIG OR SMALL.

HOW DID YOU ACCOMPLISH THEM?

HOW DID YOU FEEL AFTERWARD?

LIST THE SKILLS YOU USED.

HOW ARE YOU FEELING? CIRCLE ONE.

Date: ....

NAME THREE THINGS YOU ACCOMPLISHED TODAY, NO MATTER HOW BIG OR SMALL.

HOW DID YOU ACCOMPLISH THEM?

HOW DID YOU FEEL AFTERWARD?

LIST THE SKILLS YOU USED.

Date: ....

NAME THREE THINGS YOU ACCOMPLISHED TODAY, NO MATTER HOW BIG OR SMALL.

HOW DID YOU ACCOMPLISH THEM?

HOW DID YOU FEEL AFTERWARD?

LIST THE SKILLS YOU USED.

HOW ARE YOU FEELING? CIRCLE ONE.

Date: ....

NAME THREE THINGS YOU ACCOMPLISHED TODAY, NO MATTER HOW BIG OR SMALL.

HOW DID YOU ACCOMPLISH THEM?

HOW DID YOU FEEL AFTERWARD?

LIST THE SKILLS YOU USED.

Date: ....

NAME THREE THINGS YOU ACCOMPLISHED TODAY, NO MATTER HOW BIG OR SMALL.

HOW DID YOU ACCOMPLISH THEM?

HOW DID YOU FEEL AFTERWARD?

LIST THE SKILLS YOU USED.

HOW ARE YOU FEELING? CIRCLE ONE.

Week:

NAME THREE THINGS YOU ACCOMPLISHED TODAY, NO MATTER HOW BIG OR SMALL.

HOW DID YOU ACCOMPLISH THEM?

HOW DID YOU FEEL AFTERWARD?

LIST THE SKILLS YOU USED.

HOW ARE YOU FEELING? CIRCLE ONE.

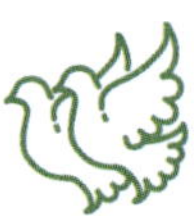

EMOTIONAL SUPPORT CHEAT SHEET

Emotional support is very important in general, but especially when it comes to mental health. Anxiety on its own is already difficult to deal with, but doing it alone is even harder. Humans are relational beings and part of this means helping and supporting each other. It's not always easy to express what kind of support you need. Here are some cheat sheets to help you convey this to others and help you understand this yourself.

EMOTIONAL SUPPORT

- Asking how someone's feeling
- Listening
- Giving hugs
- Being empathetic
- Validation

ESTEEM SUPPORT

- Pointing out someone's strengths
- Telling someone you believe in them
- Offering encouragement

INFORMATIONAL SUPPORT

- Offering advice when asked
- Sharing helpful information
- Relaying relevant anecdotes

TANGIBLE SUPPORT

- Brainstorming solutions
- Taking on a responsibility for someone else
- Bringing food or supplies over

We all need support from those who mean the most to us. Even the smallest of issues when tackled alone can feel enormous, especially when you factor in underlying anxiety and stress. Having a strong and reliable network backing you will improve your ability to cope with life's stressors on your own, so don't be afraid to ask for what you need to make yourself better.

HOW ARE YOU FEELING? CIRCLE ONE.

Now that you've seen what constitutes support, how do you feel supported? What do you respond to the best?

EMOTIONAL SUPPORT

ESTEEM SUPPORT

INFORMATIONAL SUPPORT

TANGIBLE SUPPORT

HOW ARE YOU FEELING? CIRCLE ONE.

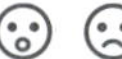   

DAILY GRATITUDE

Date:

LIST THREE THINGS YOU'RE GRATEFUL FOR.

NAME ONE THING THAT MADE YOU HAPPY TODAY.

WHO ARE YOU GRATEFUL FOR TODAY?

WHAT DO YOU LOVE ABOUT LIFE RIGHT NOW?

NAME SOMETHING YOU'RE LOOKING FORWARD TO.

DAILY GRATITUDE

Date: ....

LIST THREE THINGS YOU'RE GRATEFUL FOR.

NAME ONE THING THAT MADE YOU HAPPY TODAY.

WHO ARE YOU GRATEFUL FOR TODAY?

WHAT DO YOU LOVE ABOUT LIFE RIGHT NOW?

NAME SOMETHING YOU'RE LOOKING FORWARD TO.

HOW ARE YOU FEELING? CIRCLE ONE.

DAILY GRATITUDE

Date:

LIST THREE THINGS YOU'RE GRATEFUL FOR.

NAME ONE THING THAT MADE YOU HAPPY TODAY.

WHO ARE YOU GRATEFUL FOR TODAY?

WHAT DO YOU LOVE ABOUT LIFE RIGHT NOW?

NAME SOMETHING YOU'RE LOOKING FORWARD TO.

DAILY GRATITUDE

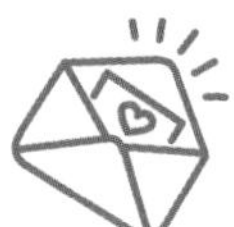

Date: ....

LIST THREE THINGS YOU'RE GRATEFUL FOR.

NAME ONE THING THAT MADE YOU HAPPY TODAY.

WHO ARE YOU GRATEFUL FOR TODAY?

WHAT DO YOU LOVE ABOUT LIFE RIGHT NOW?

NAME SOMETHING YOU'RE LOOKING FORWARD TO.

HOW ARE YOU FEELING? CIRCLE ONE.

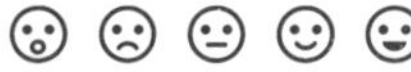

DAILY GRATITUDE

Date:

LIST THREE THINGS YOU'RE GRATEFUL FOR.

NAME ONE THING THAT MADE YOU HAPPY TODAY.

WHO ARE YOU GRATEFUL FOR TODAY?

WHAT DO YOU LOVE ABOUT LIFE RIGHT NOW?

NAME SOMETHING YOU'RE LOOKING FORWARD TO.

DAILY GRATITUDE

Date:

LIST THREE THINGS YOU'RE GRATEFUL FOR.

NAME ONE THING THAT MADE YOU HAPPY TODAY.

WHO ARE YOU GRATEFUL FOR TODAY?

WHAT DO YOU LOVE ABOUT LIFE RIGHT NOW?

NAME SOMETHING YOU'RE LOOKING FORWARD TO.

HOW ARE YOU FEELING? CIRCLE ONE.

DAILY GRATITUDE

Date:

LIST THREE THINGS YOU'RE GRATEFUL FOR.

NAME ONE THING THAT MADE YOU HAPPY TODAY.

WHO ARE YOU GRATEFUL FOR TODAY?

WHAT DO YOU LOVE ABOUT LIFE RIGHT NOW?

NAME SOMETHING YOU'RE LOOKING FORWARD TO.

DAILY GRATITUDE

Date:

LIST THREE THINGS YOU'RE GRATEFUL FOR.

NAME ONE THING THAT MADE YOU HAPPY TODAY.

WHO ARE YOU GRATEFUL FOR TODAY?

WHAT DO YOU LOVE ABOUT LIFE RIGHT NOW?

NAME SOMETHING YOU'RE LOOKING FORWARD TO.

HOW ARE YOU FEELING? CIRCLE ONE.

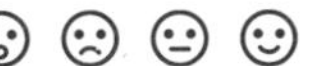

DAILY GRATITUDE

Date: ....

LIST THREE THINGS YOU'RE GRATEFUL FOR.

NAME ONE THING THAT MADE YOU HAPPY TODAY.

WHO ARE YOU GRATEFUL FOR TODAY?

WHAT DO YOU LOVE ABOUT LIFE RIGHT NOW?

NAME SOMETHING YOU'RE LOOKING FORWARD TO.

DAILY GRATITUDE

Date: ....

LIST THREE THINGS YOU'RE GRATEFUL FOR.

NAME ONE THING THAT MADE YOU HAPPY TODAY.

WHO ARE YOU GRATEFUL FOR TODAY?

WHAT DO YOU LOVE ABOUT LIFE RIGHT NOW?

NAME SOMETHING YOU'RE LOOKING FORWARD TO.

HOW ARE YOU FEELING? CIRCLE ONE.

SELF-CARE REMINDER

Self-care is a necessary component in destressing. It's your responsibility to be good to yourself and to keep track of what makes you feel happy, safe, and calm. What are some ways you use self-care?

EMOTIONAL (JOURNALING, LISTENING TO MUSIC, VENTING)

ENVIRONMENTAL (TAKING A WALK, CLEANING YOUR SPACE)

FINANCIAL (SETTING A BUDGET FOR FUN PURCHASES, PAYING DOWN DEBT WHEN POSSIBLE)

INTELLECTUAL (TRYING SOMETHING NEW, LISTENING TO AUDIOBOOKS, PLAYING STRATEGY GAMES)

OCCUPATIONAL (GETTING A CERTIFICATION, REVISING YOUR RESUME, LOOKING FOR A BETTER JOB)

PHYSICAL (WORKING OUT, EATING WELL, REMEMBERING TO TAKE PRESCRIBED MEDICATIONS)

SOCIAL (HANGING OUT WITH FRIENDS, HAVING FUN, VOLUNTEERING)

SPIRITUAL (MEDITATING, BEING KIND, BEING MINDFUL)

HOW ARE YOU FEELING? CIRCLE ONE.

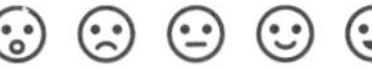

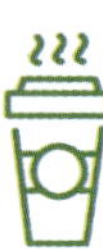

OCCUPATIONAL (GETTING A CERTIFICATION, REVISING YOUR RESUME, LOOKING FOR A BETTER JOB)

PHYSICAL (WORKING OUT, EATING WELL, REMEMBERING TO TAKE PRESCRIBED MEDICATIONS)

SOCIAL (HANGING OUT WITH FRIENDS, HAVING FUN, VOLUNTEERING)

SPIRITUAL (MEDITATING, BEING KIND, BEING MINDFUL)

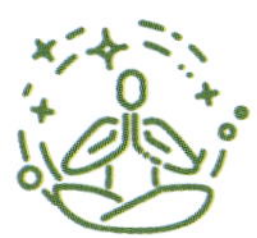

OCCUPATIONAL (GETTING A CERTIFICATION, REVISING YOUR RESUME, LOOKING FOR A BETTER JOB)

PHYSICAL (WORKING OUT, EATING WELL, REMEMBERING TO TAKE PRESCRIBED MEDICATIONS)

SOCIAL (HANGING OUT WITH FRIENDS, HAVING FUN, VOLUNTEERING)

SPIRITUAL (MEDITATING, BEING KIND, BEING MINDFUL)

HOW ARE YOU FEELING? CIRCLE ONE.

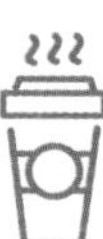

OCCUPATIONAL (GETTING A CERTIFICATION, REVISING YOUR RESUME, LOOKING FOR A BETTER JOB)

PHYSICAL (WORKING OUT, EATING WELL, REMEMBERING TO TAKE PRESCRIBED MEDICATIONS)

SOCIAL (HANGING OUT WITH FRIENDS, HAVING FUN, VOLUNTEERING)

SPIRITUAL (MEDITATING, BEING KIND, BEING MINDFUL)

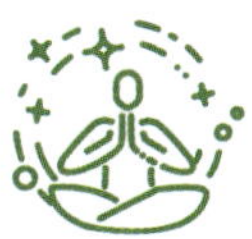

OCCUPATIONAL (GETTING A CERTIFICATION, REVISING YOUR RESUME, LOOKING FOR A BETTER JOB)

PHYSICAL (WORKING OUT, EATING WELL, REMEMBERING TO TAKE PRESCRIBED MEDICATIONS)

SOCIAL (HANGING OUT WITH FRIENDS, HAVING FUN, VOLUNTEERING)

SPIRITUAL (MEDITATING, BEING KIND, BEING MINDFUL)

HOW ARE YOU FEELING? CIRCLE ONE.

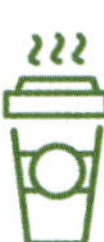

OCCUPATIONAL (GETTING A CERTIFICATION, REVISING YOUR RESUME, LOOKING FOR A BETTER JOB)

PHYSICAL (WORKING OUT, EATING WELL, REMEMBERING TO TAKE PRESCRIBED MEDICATIONS)

SOCIAL (HANGING OUT WITH FRIENDS, HAVING FUN, VOLUNTEERING)

SPIRITUAL (MEDITATING, BEING KIND, BEING MINDFUL)

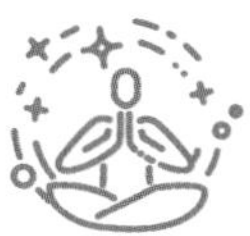

OCCUPATIONAL (GETTING A CERTIFICATION, REVISING YOUR RESUME, LOOKING FOR A BETTER JOB)

PHYSICAL (WORKING OUT, EATING WELL, REMEMBERING TO TAKE PRESCRIBED MEDICATIONS)

SOCIAL (HANGING OUT WITH FRIENDS, HAVING FUN, VOLUNTEERING)

SPIRITUAL (MEDITATING, BEING KIND, BEING MINDFUL)

HOW ARE YOU FEELING? CIRCLE ONE.

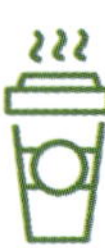

OCCUPATIONAL (GETTING A CERTIFICATION, REVISING YOUR RESUME, LOOKING FOR A BETTER JOB)

PHYSICAL (WORKING OUT, EATING WELL, REMEMBERING TO TAKE PRESCRIBED MEDICATIONS)

SOCIAL (HANGING OUT WITH FRIENDS, HAVING FUN, VOLUNTEERING)

SPIRITUAL (MEDITATING, BEING KIND, BEING MINDFUL)

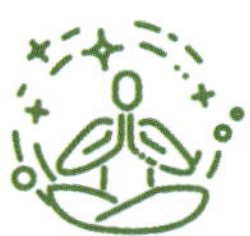

OCCUPATIONAL (GETTING A CERTIFICATION, REVISING YOUR RESUME, LOOKING FOR A BETTER JOB)

PHYSICAL (WORKING OUT, EATING WELL, REMEMBERING TO TAKE PRESCRIBED MEDICATIONS)

SOCIAL (HANGING OUT WITH FRIENDS, HAVING FUN, VOLUNTEERING)

SPIRITUAL (MEDITATING, BEING KIND, BEING MINDFUL)

HOW ARE YOU FEELING? CIRCLE ONE.

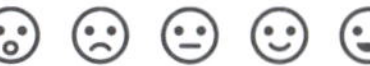

WHAT MAKES YOU THE HAPPIEST?

WHO MAKES YOU HAPPY?

WHAT'S YOUR FAVORITE FOOD?

WHAT'S YOUR FAVORITE SMELL?

WHAT'S YOUR FAVORITE SOUND?

WHAT'S YOUR FAVORITE MOVIE?

WHAT'S YOUR FAVORITE TV SHOW?

WHAT'S A GUILTY PLEASURE YOU HAVE?

WHAT'S YOUR FAVORITE JOKE?

HOW ARE YOU FEELING? CIRCLE ONE.

WHAT MAKES YOU THE HAPPIEST?

ARE YOU HAPPIER ALONE OR WITH OTHER PEOPLE?

WHICH ACTIVITY MAKES YOU THE HAPPIEST?

WHAT MAKES YOU BELLY LAUGH?

WHAT MAKES YOU SMILE?

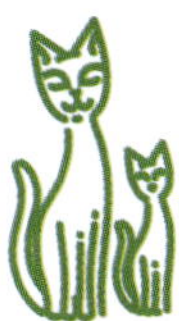

WHICH PLACE MAKES YOU THE HAPPIEST?

WHAT'S SOMETHING SMALL THAT MAKES YOU HAPPY BUT SOMETHING MOST PEOPLE DON'T NOTICE?

WHAT'S YOUR IDEA OF A GOOD DAY?

HOW ARE YOU FEELING? CIRCLE ONE.

HAPPY HABIT TRACKER

Date:

WHAT WOULD MAKE YOU HAPPY TODAY?

WHAT STEPS WILL YOU TAKE TO MAKE IT HAPPEN?

TAKE A MOMENT TO STOP AND ENJOY WHAT'S AROUND YOU. WHAT DELIGHTS YOU?

WHAT DID YOU DO TODAY TO PROMOTE HAPPINESS?

HAPPY HABIT TRACKER

Date:

WHAT WOULD MAKE YOU HAPPY TODAY?

WHAT STEPS WILL YOU TAKE TO MAKE IT HAPPEN?

TAKE A MOMENT TO STOP AND ENJOY WHAT'S AROUND YOU. WHAT DELIGHTS YOU?

WHAT DID YOU DO TODAY TO PROMOTE HAPPINESS?

HOW ARE YOU FEELING? CIRCLE ONE.

HAPPY HABIT TRACKER

Date: ....

WHAT WOULD MAKE YOU HAPPY TODAY?

WHAT STEPS WILL YOU TAKE TO MAKE IT HAPPEN?

TAKE A MOMENT TO STOP AND ENJOY WHAT'S AROUND YOU. WHAT DELIGHTS YOU?

WHAT DID YOU DO TODAY TO PROMOTE HAPPINESS?

HAPPY HABIT TRACKER

Date: ....

WHAT WOULD MAKE YOU HAPPY TODAY?

WHAT STEPS WILL YOU TAKE TO MAKE IT HAPPEN?

TAKE A MOMENT TO STOP AND ENJOY WHAT'S AROUND YOU. WHAT DELIGHTS YOU?

WHAT DID YOU DO TODAY TO PROMOTE HAPPINESS?

HOW ARE YOU FEELING? CIRCLE ONE.

HAPPY HABIT TRACKER

Date: ....

WHAT WOULD MAKE YOU HAPPY TODAY?

WHAT STEPS WILL YOU TAKE TO MAKE IT HAPPEN?

TAKE A MOMENT TO STOP AND ENJOY WHAT'S AROUND YOU. WHAT DELIGHTS YOU?

WHAT DID YOU DO TODAY TO PROMOTE HAPPINESS?

HAPPY HABIT TRACKER

Date: ....

WHAT WOULD MAKE YOU HAPPY TODAY?

WHAT STEPS WILL YOU TAKE TO MAKE IT HAPPEN?

TAKE A MOMENT TO STOP AND ENJOY WHAT'S AROUND YOU. WHAT DELIGHTS YOU?

WHAT DID YOU DO TODAY TO PROMOTE HAPPINESS?

HOW ARE YOU FEELING? CIRCLE ONE.

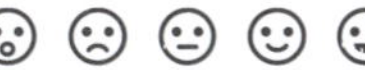

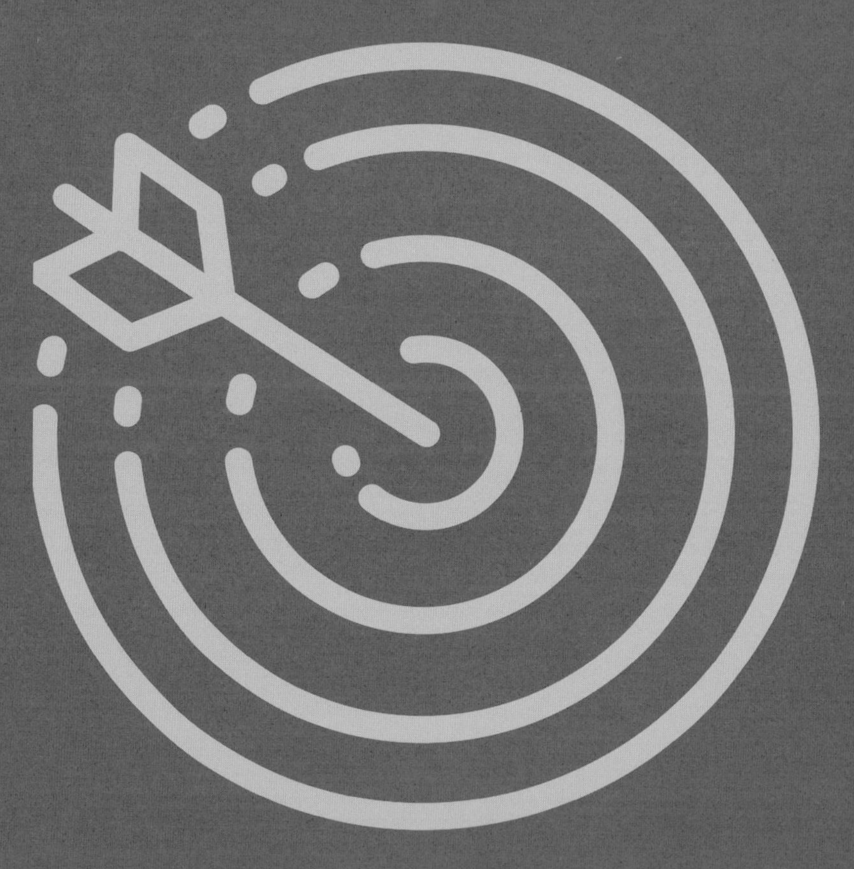

SOLUTIONS & EXERCISES

One way to manage stress is to recognize the negative thought patterns that take you there. You've documented your triggers and stressors which are starting points toward better living. From here, there's only up.

In this section, you'll learn to change your way of thinking, rewrite the stories you tell yourself, learn new coping mechanisms, and navigate through your anxiety instead of being overwhelmed by it.

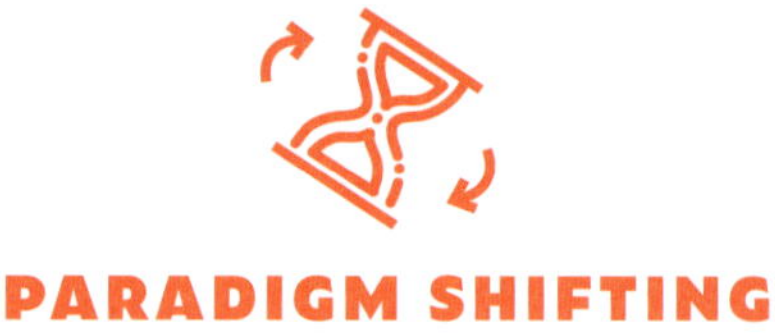

PARADIGM SHIFTING

A paradigm is a philosophical or theoretical framework of thought, similar to a story you tell yourself. Negative stories like "I can't do anything right" are setting up the framework for stress. Instead, try a new way of thinking by turning the paradigm on its head.

WRITE YOUR NEGATIVE STORY.

NOW, REFRAME YOUR STORY AS THE COMPLETE OPPOSITE.

WRITE YOUR NEGATIVE STORY.

NOW, REFRAME YOUR STORY AS THE COMPLETE OPPOSITE.

WRITE YOUR NEGATIVE STORY.

NOW, REFRAME YOUR STORY AS THE COMPLETE OPPOSITE.

WRITE YOUR NEGATIVE STORY.

NOW, REFRAME YOUR STORY AS THE COMPLETE OPPOSITE.

WHAT'S YOUR ANXIETY LEVEL RIGHT NOW? CIRCLE ONE.

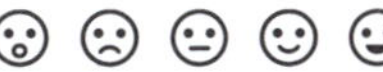

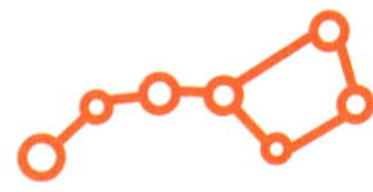

WRITE YOUR NEGATIVE STORY.

NOW, REFRAME YOUR STORY AS THE COMPLETE OPPOSITE.

WRITE YOUR NEGATIVE STORY.

NOW, REFRAME YOUR STORY AS THE COMPLETE OPPOSITE.

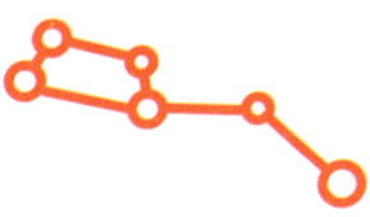

WRITE YOUR NEGATIVE STORY.

NOW, REFRAME YOUR STORY AS THE COMPLETE OPPOSITE.

WRITE YOUR NEGATIVE STORY.

NOW, REFRAME YOUR STORY AS THE COMPLETE OPPOSITE.

WHAT'S YOUR ANXIETY LEVEL RIGHT NOW? CIRCLE ONE.

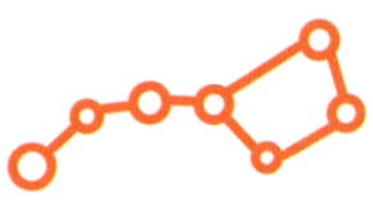

WRITE YOUR NEGATIVE STORY.

NOW, REFRAME YOUR STORY AS THE COMPLETE OPPOSITE.

WRITE YOUR NEGATIVE STORY.

NOW, REFRAME YOUR STORY AS THE COMPLETE OPPOSITE.

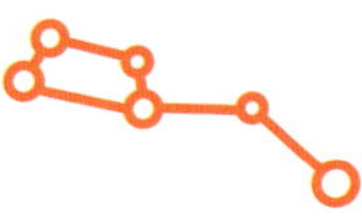

WRITE YOUR NEGATIVE STORY.

NOW, REFRAME YOUR STORY AS THE COMPLETE OPPOSITE.

WRITE YOUR NEGATIVE STORY.

NOW, REFRAME YOUR STORY AS THE COMPLETE OPPOSITE.

WHAT'S YOUR ANXIETY LEVEL RIGHT NOW? CIRCLE ONE.

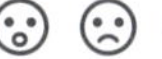   

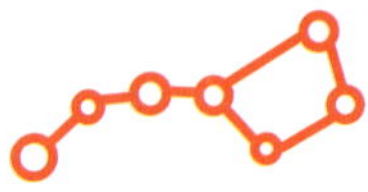

WRITE YOUR NEGATIVE STORY.

NOW, REFRAME YOUR STORY AS THE COMPLETE OPPOSITE.

WRITE YOUR NEGATIVE STORY.

NOW, REFRAME YOUR STORY AS THE COMPLETE OPPOSITE.

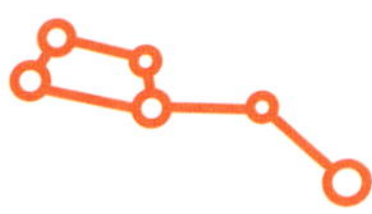

WRITE YOUR NEGATIVE STORY.

NOW, REFRAME YOUR STORY AS THE COMPLETE OPPOSITE.

WRITE YOUR NEGATIVE STORY.

NOW, REFRAME YOUR STORY AS THE COMPLETE OPPOSITE.

WHAT'S YOUR ANXIETY LEVEL RIGHT NOW? CIRCLE ONE.

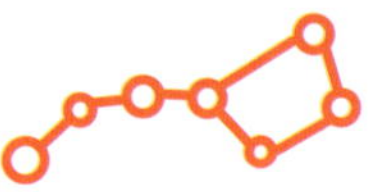

WRITE YOUR NEGATIVE STORY.

NOW, REFRAME YOUR STORY AS THE COMPLETE OPPOSITE.

WRITE YOUR NEGATIVE STORY.

NOW, REFRAME YOUR STORY AS THE COMPLETE OPPOSITE.

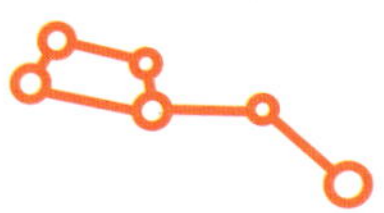

WRITE YOUR NEGATIVE STORY.

NOW, REFRAME YOUR STORY AS THE COMPLETE OPPOSITE.

WRITE YOUR NEGATIVE STORY.

NOW, REFRAME YOUR STORY AS THE COMPLETE OPPOSITE.

WHAT'S YOUR ANXIETY LEVEL RIGHT NOW? CIRCLE ONE.

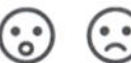   

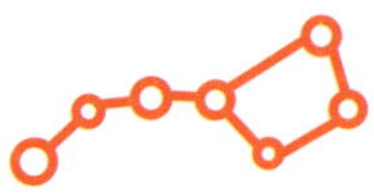

WRITE YOUR NEGATIVE STORY.

NOW, REFRAME YOUR STORY AS THE COMPLETE OPPOSITE.

WRITE YOUR NEGATIVE STORY.

NOW, REFRAME YOUR STORY AS THE COMPLETE OPPOSITE.

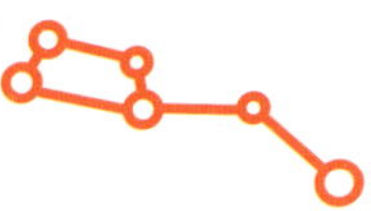

WRITE YOUR NEGATIVE STORY.

NOW, REFRAME YOUR STORY AS THE COMPLETE OPPOSITE.

WRITE YOUR NEGATIVE STORY.

NOW, REFRAME YOUR STORY AS THE COMPLETE OPPOSITE.

WHAT'S YOUR ANXIETY LEVEL RIGHT NOW? CIRCLE ONE.

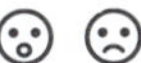   

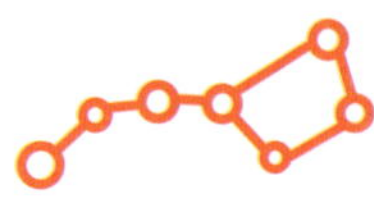

WRITE YOUR NEGATIVE STORY.

NOW, REFRAME YOUR STORY AS THE COMPLETE OPPOSITE.

WRITE YOUR NEGATIVE STORY.

NOW, REFRAME YOUR STORY AS THE COMPLETE OPPOSITE.

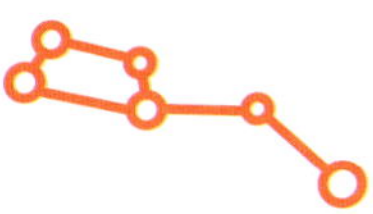

WRITE YOUR NEGATIVE STORY.

NOW, REFRAME YOUR STORY AS THE COMPLETE OPPOSITE.

WRITE YOUR NEGATIVE STORY.

NOW, REFRAME YOUR STORY AS THE COMPLETE OPPOSITE.

WHAT'S YOUR ANXIETY LEVEL RIGHT NOW? CIRCLE ONE.

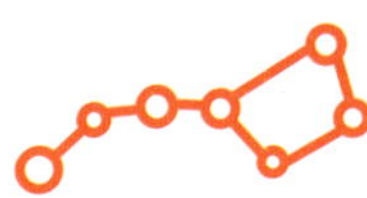

WRITE YOUR NEGATIVE STORY.

NOW, REFRAME YOUR STORY AS THE COMPLETE OPPOSITE.

WRITE YOUR NEGATIVE STORY.

NOW, REFRAME YOUR STORY AS THE COMPLETE OPPOSITE.

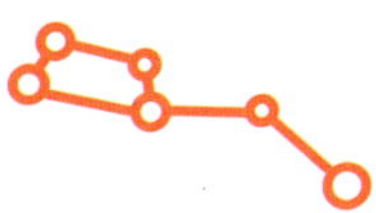

WRITE YOUR NEGATIVE STORY.

NOW, REFRAME YOUR STORY AS THE COMPLETE OPPOSITE.

WRITE YOUR NEGATIVE STORY.

NOW, REFRAME YOUR STORY AS THE COMPLETE OPPOSITE.

WHAT'S YOUR ANXIETY LEVEL RIGHT NOW? CIRCLE ONE.

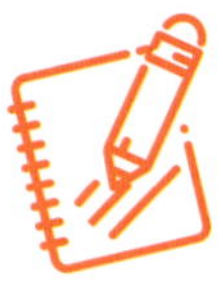

REWRITING NEGATIVE STORIES

You've listed your negative stories and their opposites. But now you'll rewrite them to better mirror reality. Instead of "I can't do anything right," you can say, "I'm feeling a lot of pressure and it's making me doubt myself." It's a separation from harmful thinking and is a more honest depiction of what's actually happening.

WHAT'S YOUR NEGATIVE STORY?

WHAT ARE YOU FEELING?

HOW CAN YOU REWRITE THIS?

WHAT'S YOUR NEGATIVE STORY?

WHAT ARE YOU FEELING?

HOW CAN YOU REWRITE THIS?

WHAT'S YOUR ANXIETY LEVEL RIGHT NOW? CIRCLE ONE.

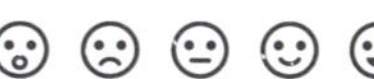

WHAT'S YOUR NEGATIVE STORY?

WHAT ARE YOU FEELING?

HOW CAN YOU REWRITE THIS?

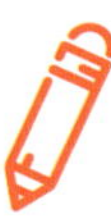

WHAT'S YOUR NEGATIVE STORY?

WHAT ARE YOU FEELING?

HOW CAN YOU REWRITE THIS?

WHAT'S YOUR ANXIETY LEVEL RIGHT NOW? CIRCLE ONE.

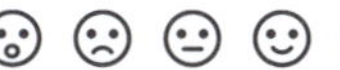

WHAT'S YOUR NEGATIVE STORY?

WHAT ARE YOU FEELING?

HOW CAN YOU REWRITE THIS?

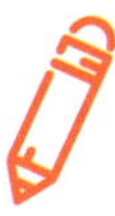

WHAT'S YOUR NEGATIVE STORY?

WHAT ARE YOU FEELING?

HOW CAN YOU REWRITE THIS?

WHAT'S YOUR ANXIETY LEVEL RIGHT NOW? CIRCLE ONE.

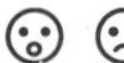   

WHAT'S YOUR NEGATIVE STORY?

WHAT ARE YOU FEELING?

HOW CAN YOU REWRITE THIS?

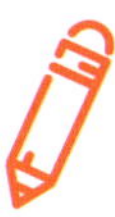

WHAT'S YOUR NEGATIVE STORY?

WHAT ARE YOU FEELING?

HOW CAN YOU REWRITE THIS?

WHAT'S YOUR ANXIETY LEVEL RIGHT NOW? CIRCLE ONE.

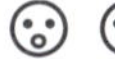   

WHAT'S YOUR NEGATIVE STORY?

WHAT ARE YOU FEELING?

HOW CAN YOU REWRITE THIS?

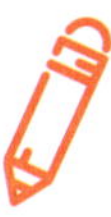

WHAT'S YOUR NEGATIVE STORY?

WHAT ARE YOU FEELING?

HOW CAN YOU REWRITE THIS?

WHAT'S YOUR ANXIETY LEVEL RIGHT NOW? CIRCLE ONE.

WHAT'S YOUR NEGATIVE STORY?

WHAT ARE YOU FEELING?

HOW CAN YOU REWRITE THIS?

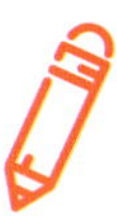

WHAT'S YOUR NEGATIVE STORY?

WHAT ARE YOU FEELING?

HOW CAN YOU REWRITE THIS?

WHAT'S YOUR ANXIETY LEVEL RIGHT NOW? CIRCLE ONE.

WHAT'S YOUR NEGATIVE STORY?

WHAT ARE YOU FEELING?

HOW CAN YOU REWRITE THIS?

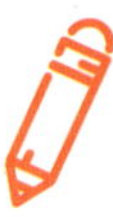

WHAT'S YOUR NEGATIVE STORY?

WHAT ARE YOU FEELING?

HOW CAN YOU REWRITE THIS?

WHAT'S YOUR ANXIETY LEVEL RIGHT NOW? CIRCLE ONE.

WHAT'S YOUR NEGATIVE STORY?

WHAT ARE YOU FEELING?

HOW CAN YOU REWRITE THIS?

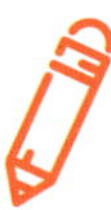

WHAT'S YOUR NEGATIVE STORY?

WHAT ARE YOU FEELING?

HOW CAN YOU REWRITE THIS?

WHAT'S YOUR ANXIETY LEVEL RIGHT NOW? CIRCLE ONE.

COPING MECHANISMS

There are two different types of healthy coping mechanisms: emotion-focused and problem-focused. The former helps with managing your feelings in stressful situations. Some examples are exercise, journaling, watching funny videos, or anything that makes you feel better. The latter is for when you want to change your situation. Some examples are making a to-do list, doing research into your problem, or asking for help.

WHAT'S WORRYING YOU?

WHICH COPING MECHANISM WILL YOU USE? WHAT WILL YOU DO?

HOW DID IT GO?

WHAT'S WORRYING YOU?

WHICH COPING MECHANISM WILL YOU USE? WHAT WILL YOU DO?

HOW DID IT GO?

WHAT'S YOUR ANXIETY LEVEL RIGHT NOW? CIRCLE ONE.

WHAT'S WORRYING YOU?

WHICH COPING MECHANISM WILL YOU USE? WHAT WILL YOU DO?

HOW DID IT GO?

WHAT'S WORRYING YOU?

WHICH COPING MECHANISM WILL YOU USE? WHAT WILL YOU DO?

HOW DID IT GO?

WHAT'S YOUR ANXIETY LEVEL RIGHT NOW? CIRCLE ONE.

WHAT'S WORRYING YOU?

WHICH COPING MECHANISM WILL YOU USE? WHAT WILL YOU DO?

HOW DID IT GO?

WHAT'S WORRYING YOU?

WHICH COPING MECHANISM WILL YOU USE? WHAT WILL YOU DO?

HOW DID IT GO?

WHAT'S YOUR ANXIETY LEVEL RIGHT NOW? CIRCLE ONE.

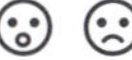   

WHAT'S WORRYING YOU?

WHICH COPING MECHANISM WILL YOU USE? WHAT WILL YOU DO?

HOW DID IT GO?

WHAT'S WORRYING YOU?

WHICH COPING MECHANISM WILL YOU USE? WHAT WILL YOU DO?

HOW DID IT GO?

WHAT'S YOUR ANXIETY LEVEL RIGHT NOW? CIRCLE ONE.

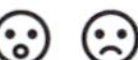   

WHAT'S WORRYING YOU?

WHICH COPING MECHANISM WILL YOU USE? WHAT WILL YOU DO?

HOW DID IT GO?

WHAT'S WORRYING YOU?

WHICH COPING MECHANISM WILL YOU USE? WHAT WILL YOU DO?

HOW DID IT GO?

WHAT'S YOUR ANXIETY LEVEL RIGHT NOW? CIRCLE ONE.

WHAT'S WORRYING YOU?

WHICH COPING MECHANISM WILL YOU USE? WHAT WILL YOU DO?

HOW DID IT GO?

WHAT'S WORRYING YOU?

WHICH COPING MECHANISM WILL YOU USE? WHAT WILL YOU DO?

HOW DID IT GO?

WHAT'S YOUR ANXIETY LEVEL RIGHT NOW? CIRCLE ONE.

WHAT'S WORRYING YOU?

WHICH COPING MECHANISM WILL YOU USE? WHAT WILL YOU DO?

HOW DID IT GO?

WHAT'S WORRYING YOU?

WHICH COPING MECHANISM WILL YOU USE? WHAT WILL YOU DO?

HOW DID IT GO?

WHAT'S YOUR ANXIETY LEVEL RIGHT NOW? CIRCLE ONE.

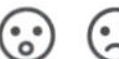   

WHAT'S WORRYING YOU?

WHICH COPING MECHANISM WILL YOU USE? WHAT WILL YOU DO?

HOW DID IT GO?

WHAT'S WORRYING YOU?

WHICH COPING MECHANISM WILL YOU USE? WHAT WILL YOU DO?

HOW DID IT GO?

WHAT'S YOUR ANXIETY LEVEL RIGHT NOW? CIRCLE ONE.

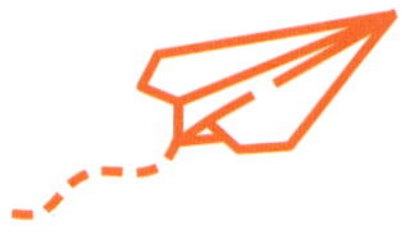

NAVIGATING THE WORLD WITH THE NEW YOU

You're a different person than when you started this journal. After all this reflection, it's time to put your new knowledge and skills to the test and explore what your life will look like with your anxiety better under control.

HOW WOULD YOU DESCRIBE YOURSELF PRE-JOURNAL?

HOW WOULD YOU DESCRIBE YOURSELF NOW?

WHO DO YOU HOPE TO BE IN THE FUTURE?

Week of: ....

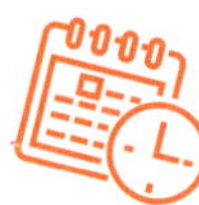

WHAT ARE YOUR GOALS FOR THIS WEEK?

HAVE YOU MADE TIME FOR SELF-CARE? IF SO, WHAT DID YOU DO?

WHICH COPING MECHANISM(S) ARE YOU USING, IF ANY?

WHICH NEGATIVE STORIES DID YOU REWRITE?

HOW WOULD YOU RATE YOUR STRESS OVERALL?

Week of: ....

WHAT ARE YOUR GOALS FOR THIS WEEK?

HAVE YOU MADE TIME FOR SELF-CARE? IF SO, WHAT DID YOU DO?

WHICH COPING MECHANISM(S) ARE YOU USING, IF ANY?

WHICH NEGATIVE STORIES DID YOU REWRITE?

Week of: ....

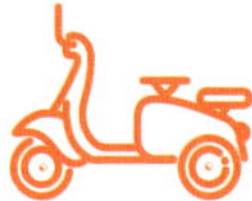

WHAT ARE YOUR GOALS FOR THIS WEEK?

HAVE YOU MADE TIME FOR SELF-CARE? IF SO, WHAT DID YOU DO?

WHICH COPING MECHANISM(S) ARE YOU USING, IF ANY?

WHICH NEGATIVE STORIES DID YOU REWRITE?

HOW WOULD YOU RATE YOUR STRESS OVERALL?

Week of: ....

WHAT ARE YOUR GOALS FOR THIS WEEK?

HAVE YOU MADE TIME FOR SELF-CARE? IF SO, WHAT DID YOU DO?

WHICH COPING MECHANISM(S) ARE YOU USING, IF ANY?

WHICH NEGATIVE STORIES DID YOU REWRITE?

Week of: ....

WHAT ARE YOUR GOALS FOR THIS WEEK?

HAVE YOU MADE TIME FOR SELF-CARE? IF SO, WHAT DID YOU DO?

WHICH COPING MECHANISM(S) ARE YOU USING, IF ANY?

WHICH NEGATIVE STORIES DID YOU REWRITE?

HOW WOULD YOU RATE YOUR STRESS OVERALL?

Week of: ....

WHAT ARE YOUR GOALS FOR THIS WEEK?

HAVE YOU MADE TIME FOR SELF-CARE? IF SO, WHAT DID YOU DO?

WHICH COPING MECHANISM(S) ARE YOU USING, IF ANY?

WHICH NEGATIVE STORIES DID YOU REWRITE?

Week of: ....

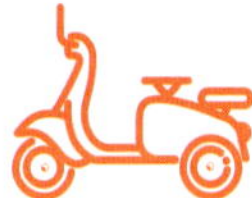

WHAT ARE YOUR GOALS FOR THIS WEEK?

HAVE YOU MADE TIME FOR SELF-CARE? IF SO, WHAT DID YOU DO?

WHICH COPING MECHANISM(S) ARE YOU USING, IF ANY?

WHICH NEGATIVE STORIES DID YOU REWRITE?

HOW WOULD YOU RATE YOUR STRESS OVERALL?

Week of:

WHAT ARE YOUR GOALS FOR THIS WEEK?

HAVE YOU MADE TIME FOR SELF-CARE? IF SO, WHAT DID YOU DO?

WHICH COPING MECHANISM(S) ARE YOU USING, IF ANY?

WHICH NEGATIVE STORIES DID YOU REWRITE?

Week of: ....

WHAT ARE YOUR GOALS FOR THIS WEEK?

HAVE YOU MADE TIME FOR SELF-CARE? IF SO, WHAT DID YOU DO?

WHICH COPING MECHANISM(S) ARE YOU USING, IF ANY?

WHICH NEGATIVE STORIES DID YOU REWRITE?

HOW WOULD YOU RATE YOUR STRESS OVERALL?

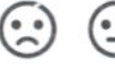  

Week of: ....

WHAT ARE YOUR GOALS FOR THIS WEEK?

HAVE YOU MADE TIME FOR SELF-CARE? IF SO, WHAT DID YOU DO?

WHICH COPING MECHANISM(S) ARE YOU USING, IF ANY?

WHICH NEGATIVE STORIES DID YOU REWRITE?

Week of: ....

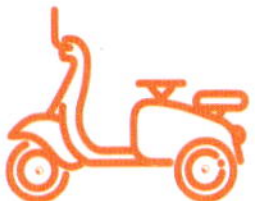

WHAT ARE YOUR GOALS FOR THIS WEEK?

HAVE YOU MADE TIME FOR SELF-CARE? IF SO, WHAT DID YOU DO?

WHICH COPING MECHANISM(S) ARE YOU USING, IF ANY?

WHICH NEGATIVE STORIES DID YOU REWRITE?

HOW WOULD YOU RATE YOUR STRESS OVERALL?

😮 ☹ 😐 🙂 😃

Week of:

WHAT ARE YOUR GOALS FOR THIS WEEK?

HAVE YOU MADE TIME FOR SELF-CARE? IF SO, WHAT DID YOU DO?

WHICH COPING MECHANISM(S) ARE YOU USING, IF ANY?

WHICH NEGATIVE STORIES DID YOU REWRITE?

Week of:

WHAT ARE YOUR GOALS FOR THIS WEEK?

HAVE YOU MADE TIME FOR SELF-CARE? IF SO, WHAT DID YOU DO?

WHICH COPING MECHANISM(S) ARE YOU USING, IF ANY?

WHICH NEGATIVE STORIES DID YOU REWRITE?

HOW WOULD YOU RATE YOUR STRESS OVERALL?

Week of:

WHAT ARE YOUR GOALS FOR THIS WEEK?

HAVE YOU MADE TIME FOR SELF-CARE? IF SO, WHAT DID YOU DO?

WHICH COPING MECHANISM(S) ARE YOU USING, IF ANY?

WHICH NEGATIVE STORIES DID YOU REWRITE?

Week of: ....

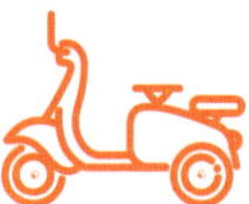

WHAT ARE YOUR GOALS FOR THIS WEEK?

HAVE YOU MADE TIME FOR SELF-CARE? IF SO, WHAT DID YOU DO?

WHICH COPING MECHANISM(S) ARE YOU USING, IF ANY?

WHICH NEGATIVE STORIES DID YOU REWRITE?

HOW WOULD YOU RATE YOUR STRESS OVERALL?

Week of:

WHAT ARE YOUR GOALS FOR THIS WEEK?

HAVE YOU MADE TIME FOR SELF-CARE? IF SO, WHAT DID YOU DO?

WHICH COPING MECHANISM(S) ARE YOU USING, IF ANY?

WHICH NEGATIVE STORIES DID YOU REWRITE?

Week of:

WHAT ARE YOUR GOALS FOR THIS WEEK?

HAVE YOU MADE TIME FOR SELF-CARE? IF SO, WHAT DID YOU DO?

WHICH COPING MECHANISM(S) ARE YOU USING, IF ANY?

WHICH NEGATIVE STORIES DID YOU REWRITE?

HOW WOULD YOU RATE YOUR STRESS OVERALL?

Week of:

WHAT ARE YOUR GOALS FOR THIS WEEK?

HAVE YOU MADE TIME FOR SELF-CARE? IF SO, WHAT DID YOU DO?

WHICH COPING MECHANISM(S) ARE YOU USING, IF ANY?

WHICH NEGATIVE STORIES DID YOU REWRITE?

Week of:

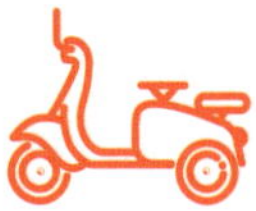

WHAT ARE YOUR GOALS FOR THIS WEEK?

HAVE YOU MADE TIME FOR SELF-CARE? IF SO, WHAT DID YOU DO?

WHICH COPING MECHANISM(S) ARE YOU USING, IF ANY?

WHICH NEGATIVE STORIES DID YOU REWRITE?

HOW WOULD YOU RATE YOUR STRESS OVERALL?

😮 ☹ 😐 🙂 😃

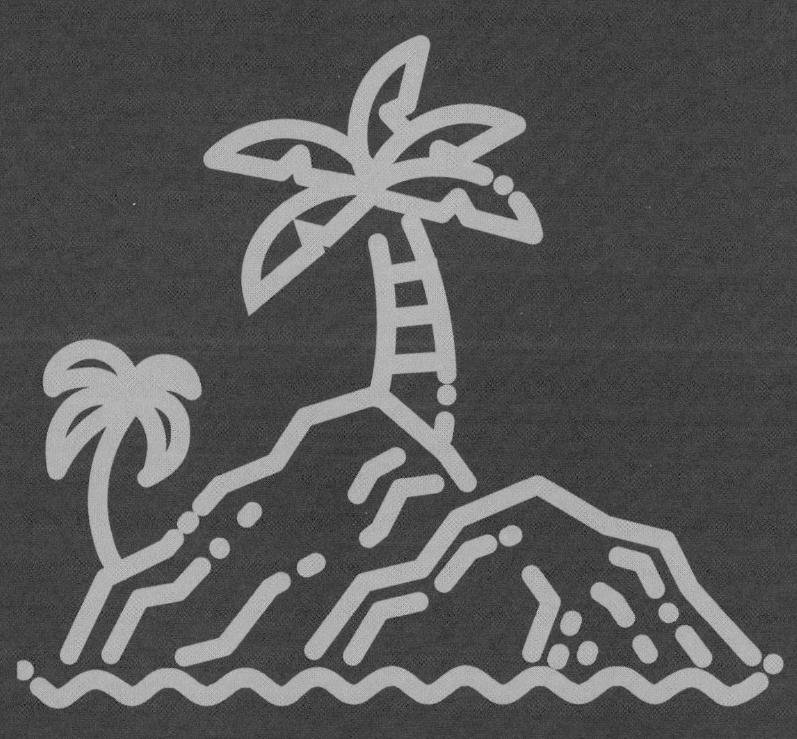

POST-JOURNAL JOURNEY

You've done the work, you've reflected, and now you're on the other side. You have the tools to manage your anxiety and live your life a little more stress free. In this section, you'll check in with yourself, reflect on your feelings now, and track your wellness. From here and beyond, it gets easier.

HOW DO YOU FEEL NOW?

RATE YOUR STRESS LEVEL.

HOW'S LIFE GOING?

WHAT NEW COPING MECHANISMS HAVE YOU IMPLEMENTED?

WHAT ARE YOU GRATEFUL FOR NOW?

DID YOU REACH YOUR GOALS FROM THE BEGINNING OF YOUR JOURNEY? WHICH ONES?

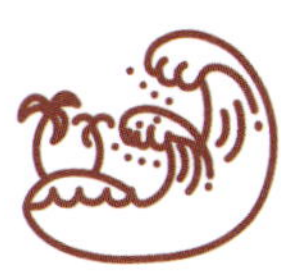

WHAT HAVE YOU LEARNED ABOUT YOURSELF?

HOW HAVE YOU CHANGED OVER THE COURSE OF THIS JOURNAL?

HOW DO YOU FEEL NOW?

WHAT'S YOUR ANXIETY LEVEL RIGHT NOW? CIRCLE ONE.

MONTHLY CHECK-IN

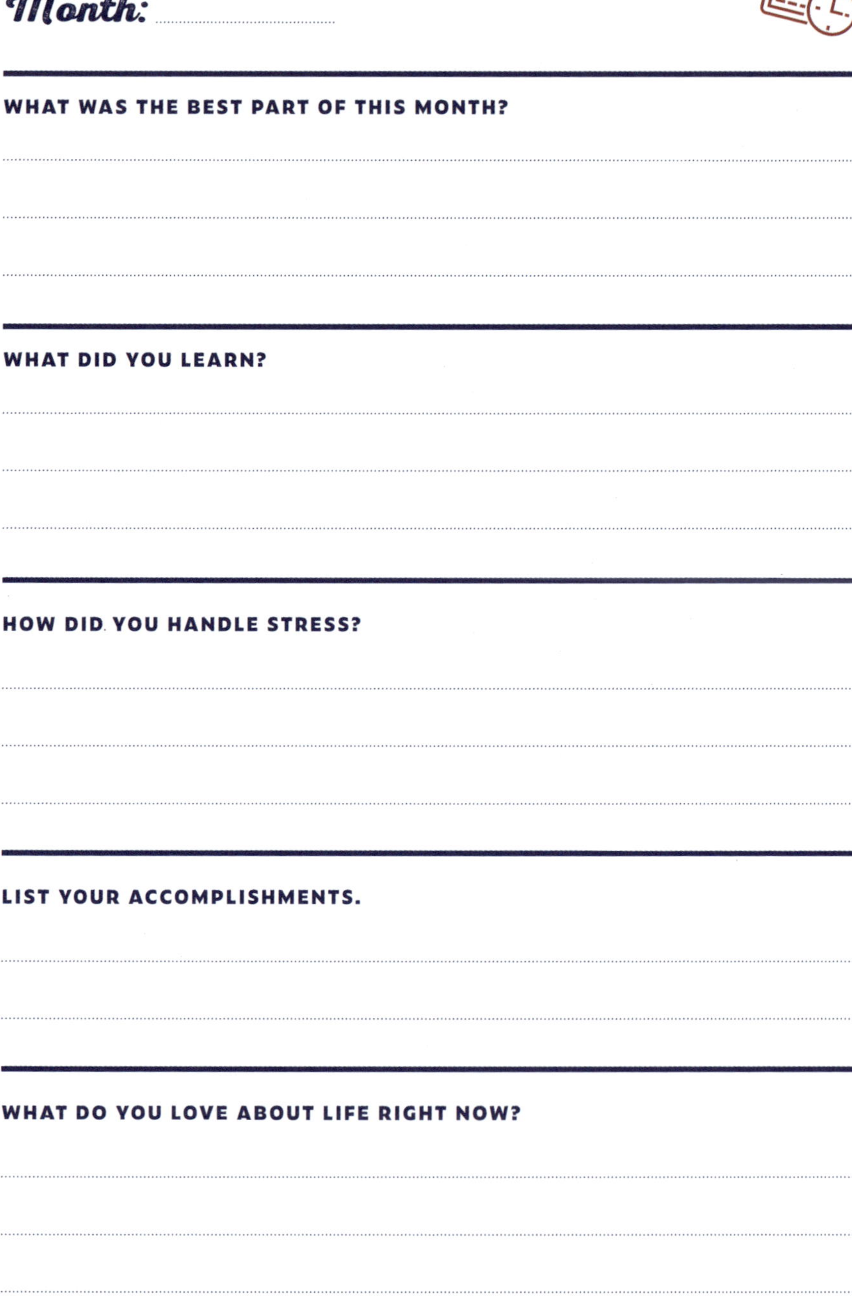

Month: ....

WHAT WAS THE BEST PART OF THIS MONTH?

WHAT DID YOU LEARN?

HOW DID YOU HANDLE STRESS?

LIST YOUR ACCOMPLISHMENTS.

WHAT DO YOU LOVE ABOUT LIFE RIGHT NOW?

MONTHLY CHECK-IN

Month:

WHAT WAS THE BEST PART OF THIS MONTH?

WHAT DID YOU LEARN?

HOW DID YOU HANDLE STRESS?

LIST YOUR ACCOMPLISHMENTS.

WHAT DO YOU LOVE ABOUT LIFE RIGHT NOW?

WHAT'S YOUR ANXIETY LEVEL RIGHT NOW? CIRCLE ONE.

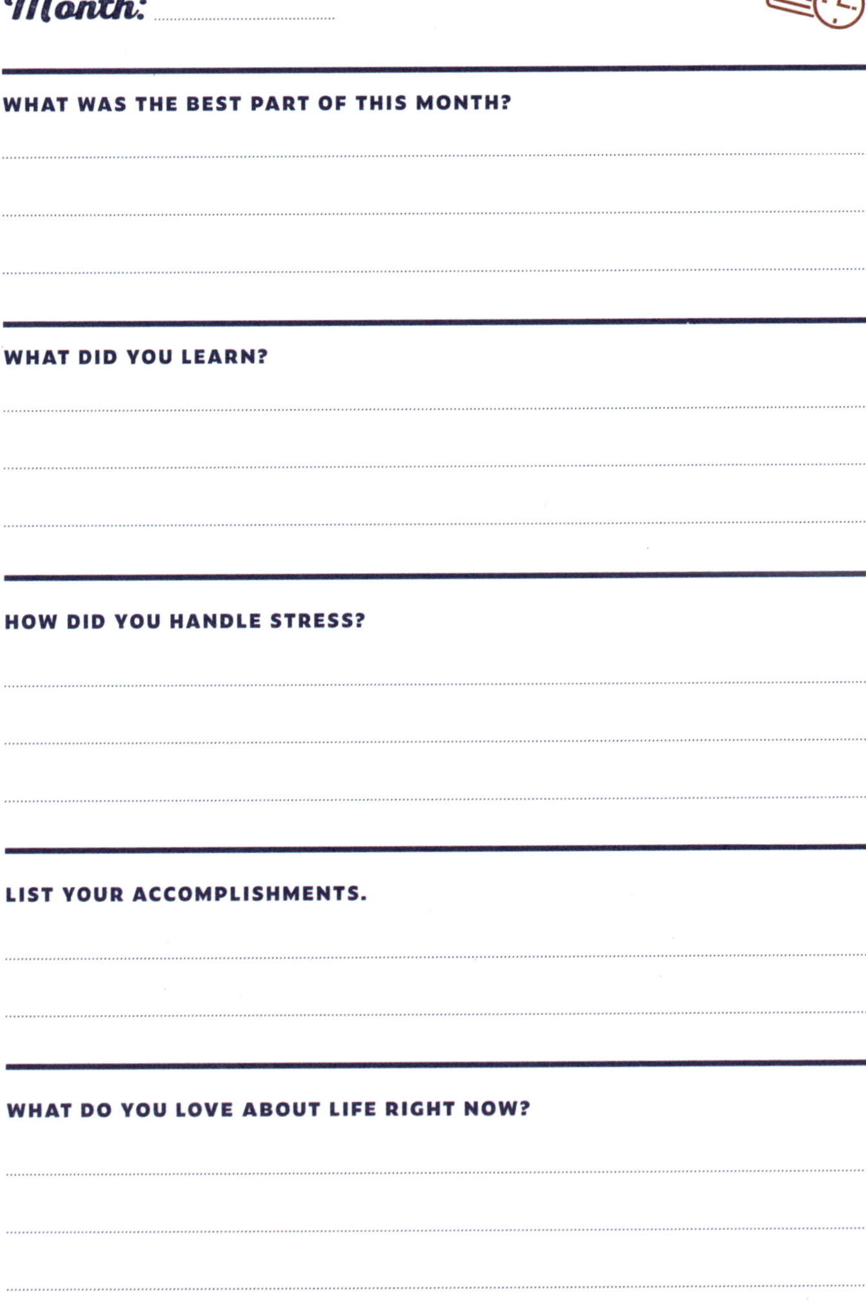

MONTHLY CHECK-IN

Month: ....

WHAT WAS THE BEST PART OF THIS MONTH?

WHAT DID YOU LEARN?

HOW DID YOU HANDLE STRESS?

LIST YOUR ACCOMPLISHMENTS.

WHAT DO YOU LOVE ABOUT LIFE RIGHT NOW?

MONTHLY CHECK-IN

Month: ....

WHAT WAS THE BEST PART OF THIS MONTH?

WHAT DID YOU LEARN?

HOW DID YOU HANDLE STRESS?

LIST YOUR ACCOMPLISHMENTS.

WHAT DO YOU LOVE ABOUT LIFE RIGHT NOW?

WHAT'S YOUR ANXIETY LEVEL RIGHT NOW? CIRCLE ONE.

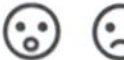   

MONTHLY CHECK-IN

Month: ....

WHAT WAS THE BEST PART OF THIS MONTH?

WHAT DID YOU LEARN?

HOW DID YOU HANDLE STRESS?

LIST YOUR ACCOMPLISHMENTS.

WHAT DO YOU LOVE ABOUT LIFE RIGHT NOW?

MONTHLY CHECK-IN

Month: ....

WHAT WAS THE BEST PART OF THIS MONTH?

WHAT DID YOU LEARN?

HOW DID YOU HANDLE STRESS?

LIST YOUR ACCOMPLISHMENTS.

WHAT DO YOU LOVE ABOUT LIFE RIGHT NOW?

WHAT'S YOUR ANXIETY LEVEL RIGHT NOW? CIRCLE ONE.

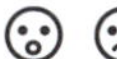   

MONTHLY CHECK-IN

Month:

WHAT WAS THE BEST PART OF THIS MONTH?

WHAT DID YOU LEARN?

HOW DID YOU HANDLE STRESS?

LIST YOUR ACCOMPLISHMENTS.

WHAT DO YOU LOVE ABOUT LIFE RIGHT NOW?

MONTHLY CHECK-IN

Month: ....

WHAT WAS THE BEST PART OF THIS MONTH?

WHAT DID YOU LEARN?

HOW DID YOU HANDLE STRESS?

LIST YOUR ACCOMPLISHMENTS.

WHAT DO YOU LOVE ABOUT LIFE RIGHT NOW?

WHAT'S YOUR ANXIETY LEVEL RIGHT NOW? CIRCLE ONE.

MONTHLY CHECK-IN

Month: ....

WHAT WAS THE BEST PART OF THIS MONTH?

WHAT DID YOU LEARN?

HOW DID YOU HANDLE STRESS?

LIST YOUR ACCOMPLISHMENTS.

WHAT DO YOU LOVE ABOUT LIFE RIGHT NOW?

MONTHLY CHECK-IN

Month: ....

WHAT WAS THE BEST PART OF THIS MONTH?

WHAT DID YOU LEARN?

HOW DID YOU HANDLE STRESS?

LIST YOUR ACCOMPLISHMENTS.

WHAT DO YOU LOVE ABOUT LIFE RIGHT NOW?

WHAT'S YOUR ANXIETY LEVEL RIGHT NOW? CIRCLE ONE.

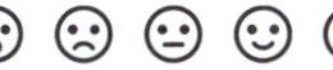

MONTHLY CHECK-IN

Month: ....

WHAT WAS THE BEST PART OF THIS MONTH?

WHAT DID YOU LEARN?

HOW DID YOU HANDLE STRESS?

LIST YOUR ACCOMPLISHMENTS.

WHAT DO YOU LOVE ABOUT LIFE RIGHT NOW?

MONTHLY CHECK-IN

Month: ....

WHAT WAS THE BEST PART OF THIS MONTH?

WHAT DID YOU LEARN?

HOW DID YOU HANDLE STRESS?

LIST YOUR ACCOMPLISHMENTS.

WHAT DO YOU LOVE ABOUT LIFE RIGHT NOW?

WHAT'S YOUR ANXIETY LEVEL RIGHT NOW? CIRCLE ONE.

WELLNESS TRACKER

Date: ....

IRRITABILITY

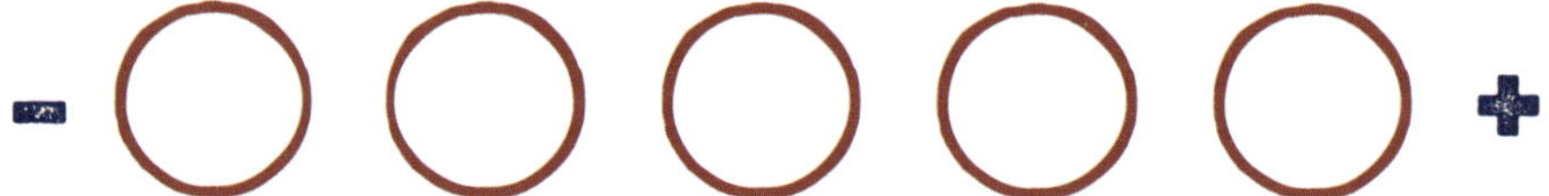

QUALITY OF SLEEP

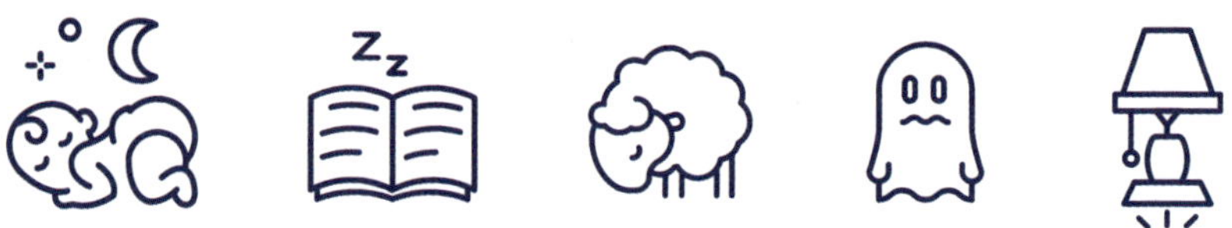

WATER INTAKE

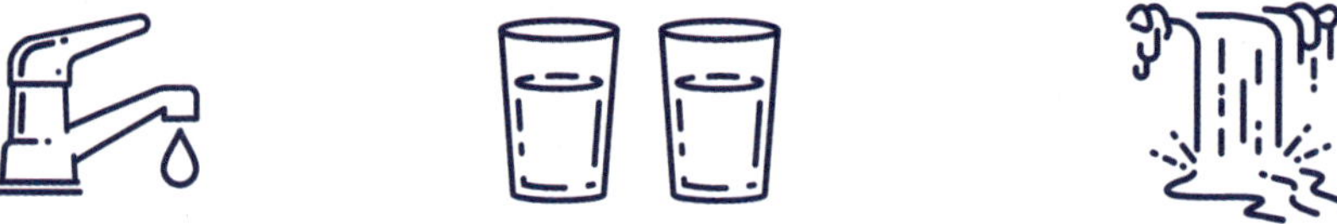

ANXIETY

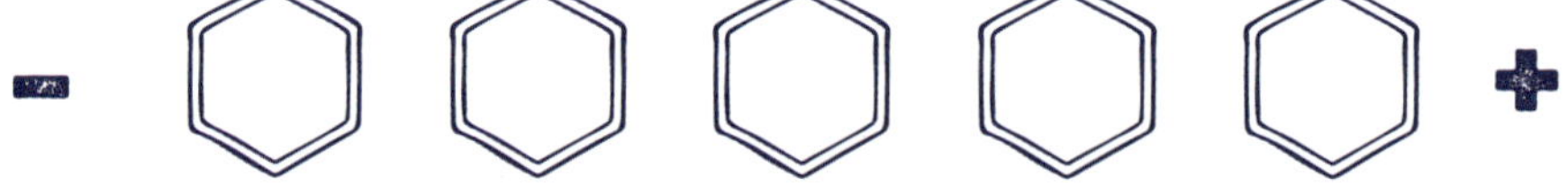

PHYSICAL ACTIVITY											
-	1	2	3	4	5	6	7	8	9	10	+

HOURS SLEPT											
-	1	2	3	4	5	6	7	8	9	10	+

HAPPY HABIT TRACKER							
HABIT TO TRACK:	S	M	T	W	TH	F	S

MEDICATION	HOW MUCH	DAY/TIME

HOW ARE YOU FEELING? CIRCLE ONE.

WELLNESS TRACKER

Date: ....

IRRITABILITY

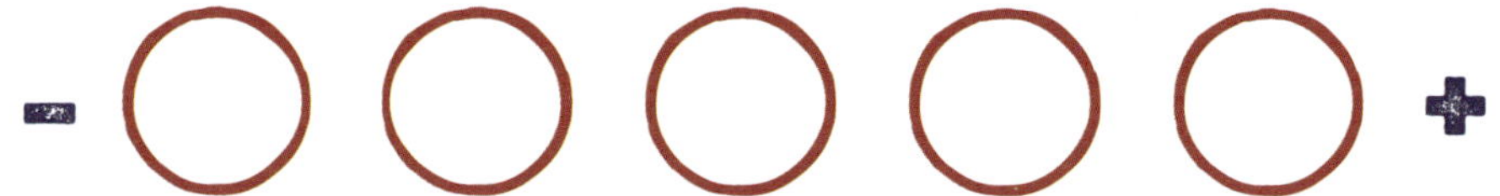

QUALITY OF SLEEP

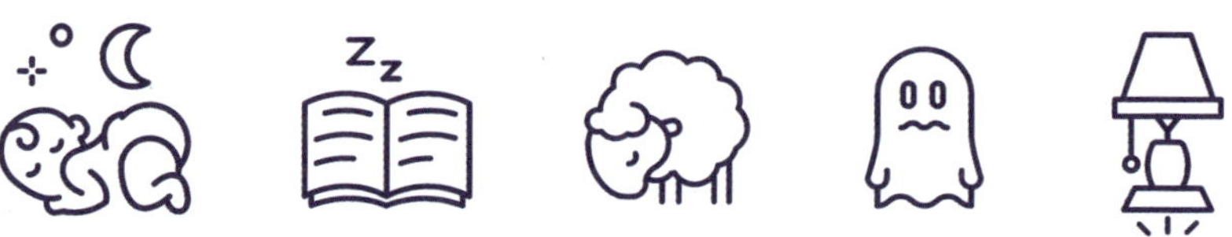

WATER INTAKE

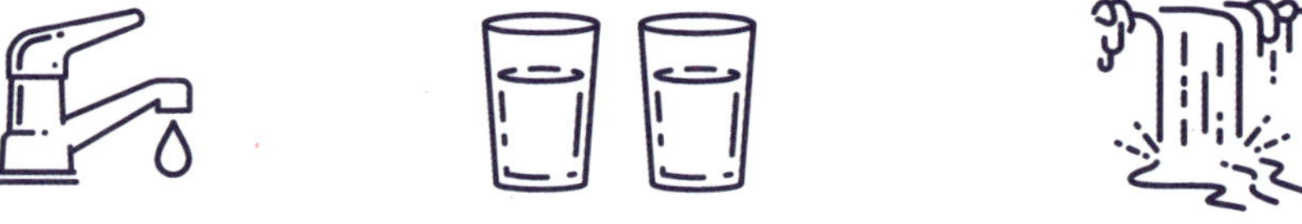

ANXIETY

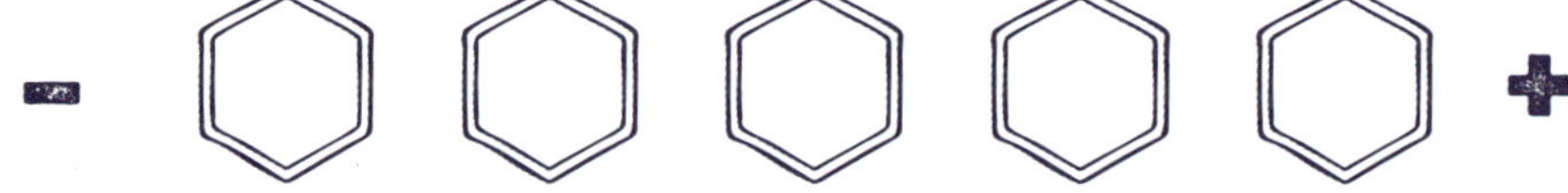

PHYSICAL ACTIVITY											
-	1	2	3	4	5	6	7	8	9	10	+

HOURS SLEPT											
-	1	2	3	4	5	6	7	8	9	10	+

HAPPY HABIT TRACKER							
HABIT TO TRACK:	S	M	T	W	TH	F	S

MEDICATION	HOW MUCH	DAY/TIME

HOW ARE YOU FEELING? CIRCLE ONE.

WELLNESS TRACKER

Date: ....

IRRITABILITY

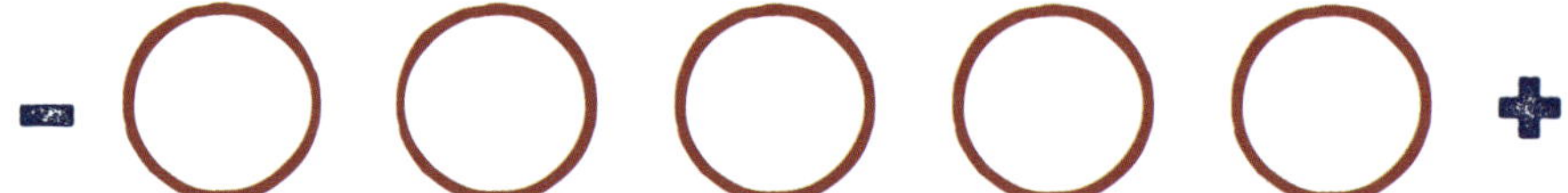

QUALITY OF SLEEP

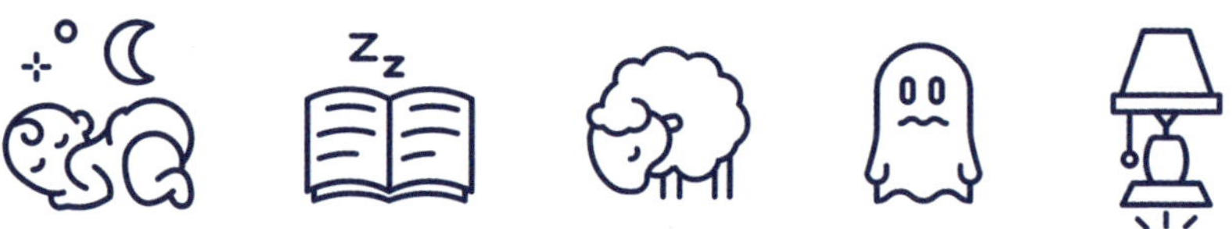

WATER INTAKE

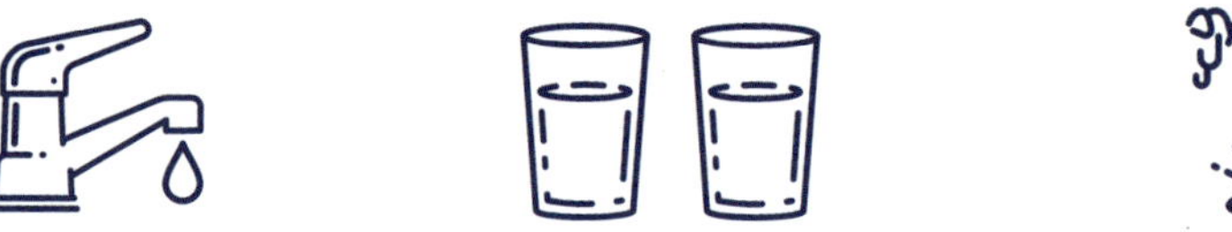

ANXIETY

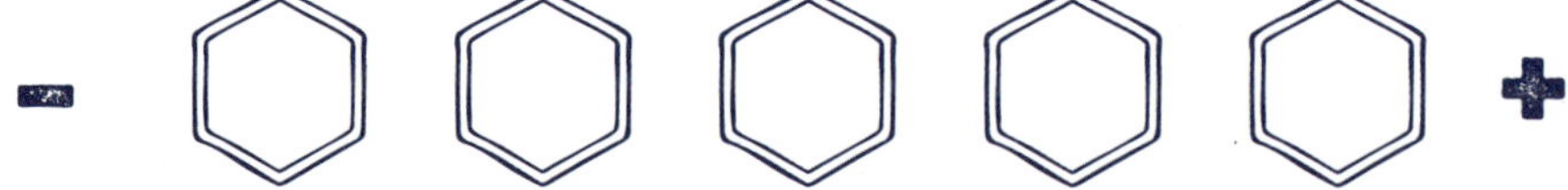

PHYSICAL ACTIVITY											
-	1	2	3	4	5	6	7	8	9	10	+

HOURS SLEPT											
-	1	2	3	4	5	6	7	8	9	10	+

HAPPY HABIT TRACKER							
HABIT TO TRACK:	S	M	T	W	TH	F	S

MEDICATION	HOW MUCH	DAY/TIME

HOW ARE YOU FEELING? CIRCLE ONE.

WELLNESS TRACKER

Date: ....

IRRITABILITY

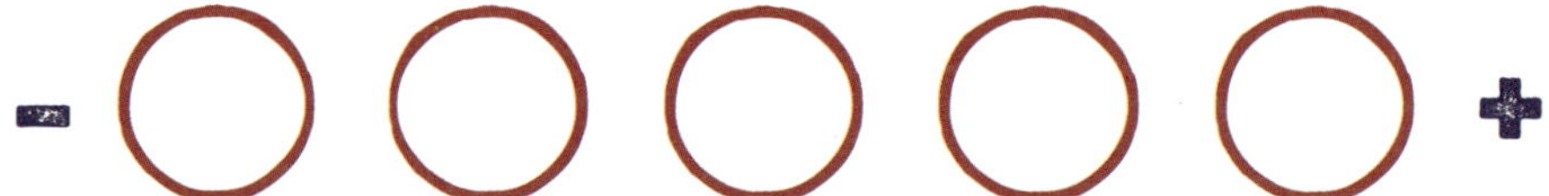

QUALITY OF SLEEP

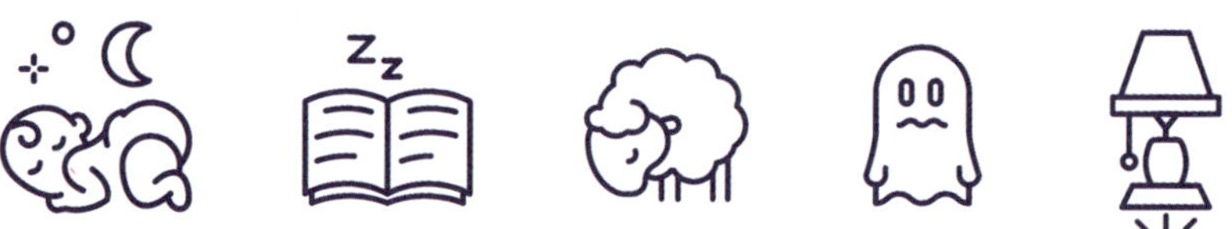

WATER INTAKE

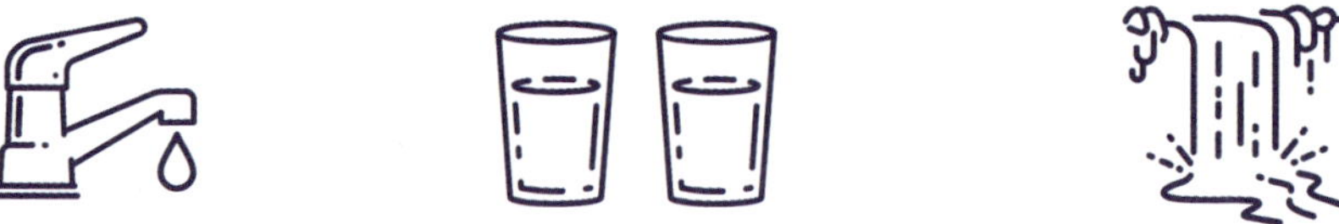

ANXIETY

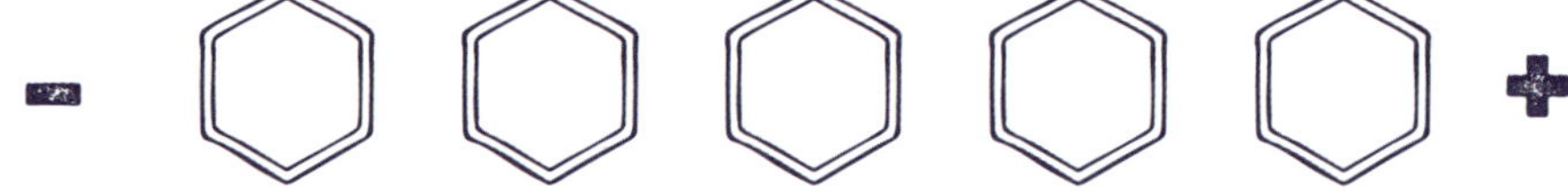

PHYSICAL ACTIVITY											
-	1	2	3	4	5	6	7	8	9	10	+

HOURS SLEPT											
-	1	2	3	4	5	6	7	8	9	10	+

HAPPY HABIT TRACKER

HABIT TO TRACK:	S	M	T	W	TH	F	S

MEDICATION	HOW MUCH	DAY/TIME

HOW ARE YOU FEELING? CIRCLE ONE.

😮 ☹ 😐 🙂 😃

Quarto

Contains content originally published as *The Anti-Anxiety Journal*, 2023, by Chartwell Books.

This edition published in 2026 by Chartwell Books,
an imprint of The Quarto Group
142 West 36th Street, 4th Floor
New York, NY 10018 USA
T (212) 779-4972
www.Quarto.com

10 9 8 7 6 5 4 3 2 1
Chartwell titles are also available at discount for retail, wholesale, promotional, and bulk purchase. For details, contact the Special Sales Manager by email at specialsales@quarto.com or by mail at The Quarto Group, Attn: Special Sales Manager, 100 Cummings Center Suite 265D, Beverly, MA 01915, USA.

ISBN: 978-0-7858-4903-2
Publisher: Wendy Friedman
Publishing Director: Meredith Mennitt
Publisher: Rage Kindelsperger
Creative Director: Laura Drew
Managing Editor: Cara Donaldson
Interior Design: Beth Middleworth
Page Layout: James Kegley
Cover: Angelika Piwowarczyk

Printed in Malaysia, PC1025

EEA Representation, WTS Tax d.o.o.,
Žanova ulica 3, 4000 Kranj, Slovenia.
www.wts-tax.si